SI KING AND DAVE MYERS

THE HAIRY *Dieters*

EAT WELL EVERY DAY

CONTENTS

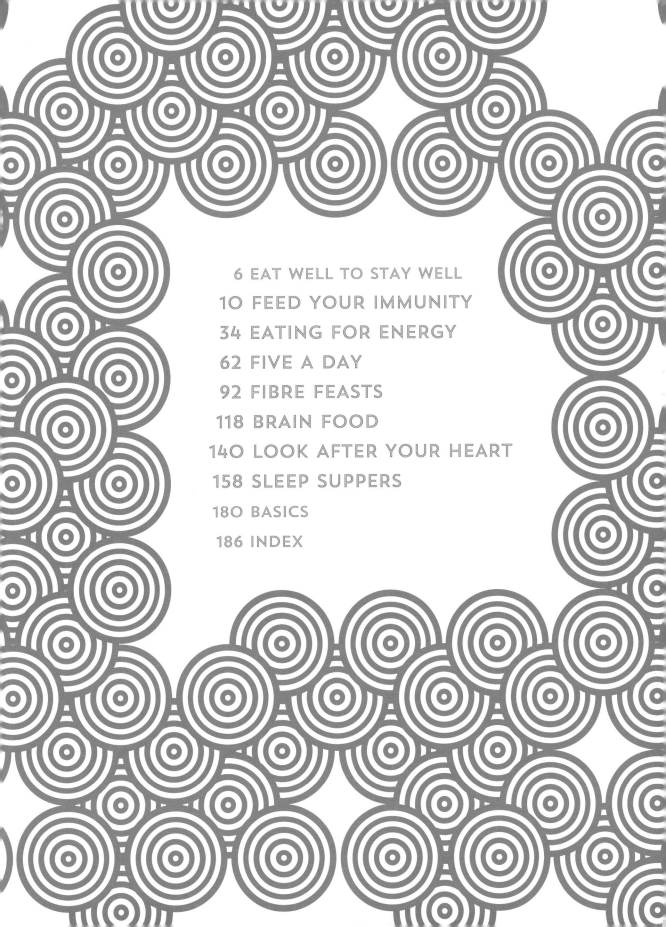

EAT WELL TO STAY WELL

Would you believe that it's been twenty years since we started out on our Hairy Bikers' adventure? And in that time, we've learned so much about food and eating well, particularly since launching our 'Hairy Dieters' series in 2012. As proper foodies and keen cooks, it hasn't always been easy to keep ourselves on the straight and narrow, but we've worked hard and we've achieved our goal weights. Now, in our different ways, we're looking to stay on track and keep fit and healthy for the long term.

We know we're not alone in sometimes wanting to splash out on a special meal or just enjoy a fry-up in the local caff — and we'll be continuing to do that from time to time — but it's a question of balance, particularly as you get older. Most nutrition and diet experts say that it's what you do 80 per cent of the time that really matters. You can cope with the occasional lapse or treat, but your day-to-day menu should focus on the good stuff if you want to stay healthy.

This makes total sense to us and it's something we can relate to as keen motorcyclists. We've travelled the world on our trusty bikes and sometimes we've found ourselves in places where we've had no option but to fill up with bad-quality petrol — and the engines don't like it. You can get away with it once in a while, but too much and the bike gives up the ghost. We reckon it's a bit like that with our bodies. Bad fuel doesn't provide the nourishment we need for our brain, our heart and our gut, and our health suffers.

With the team, we looked at coming up with recipes to maximise well-being in seven different categories — strengthening immunity and gut health, maintaining energy, reaching — or exceeding — that five-a-day goal, increasing our intake of fibre, boosting brain power, looking after the heart and aiding sleep. We listed ingredients that we know help to achieve these goals and then the job was to create recipes that were not only tasty but also ticked these seven health boxes.

We've organised the recipes into the different chapters focused on various health needs, but obviously many of the dishes are great for more than one health reason. For instance, the leek and Jerusalem artichoke soup on page 14 is a good immune booster but also contains a third of your daily fibre needs, so it's a win-win. The tasty little chia seed puddings on page 96 make a delicious breakfast and as they are served with kiwis, which are believed to aid restful sleep, you might also like to try them as a bedtime snack.

As we worked, we've learned what foods have the most nutritional value — the ones that give you more bangs for your buck in other words. For instance, nuts are real little powerhouses. They're fantastic for your immune system and gut health, great for energy and are good for brain health and your heart — and walnuts may aid sleep. Dark leafy greens are another super-food. They're packed with vitamins and minerals and are good for your brain, energy and gut.

As always, we've made sure the recipes in this book are really tasty, but that they have a purpose too. While we have included calorie counts, we've focused more on helping you keep your body a very healthy machine rather than simply on weight loss.

We believe that the aim, above all, is to be in tip-top condition health-wise, while not sacrificing one of life's greatest pleasures — enjoying good food.

Dave I've had the additional challenge of cancer during this last year and now I'm looking to recuperate while continuing chemo. I'm working hard to replace what my illness and treatment have taken from my body, and I'm determined to practise what I preach, as all this has brought home to me just how precious life is.

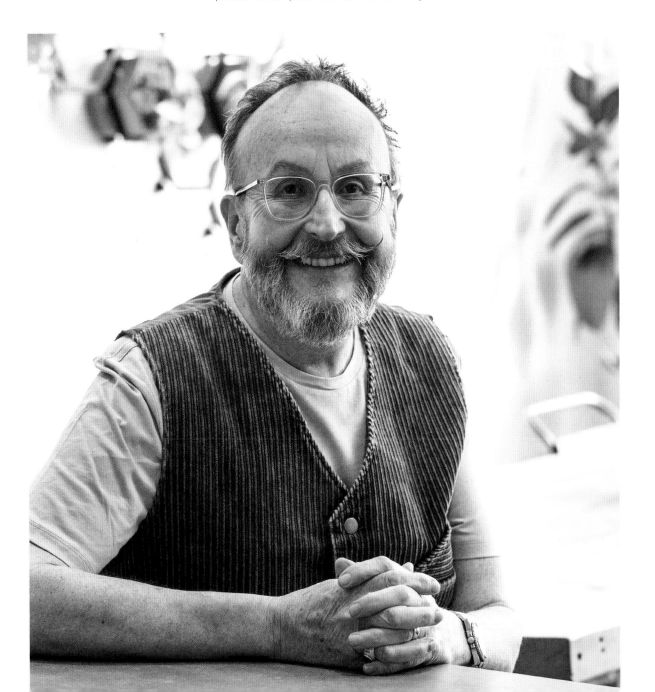

Si. My interest in good food goes back a long way. When I was growing up, Mam was always very aware of the benefits of certain foods – she used to say, 'You might not get kissed if you eat garlic, but you'll stay healthy' . That mindset has stayed with me and I firmly believe in the importance of eating well to stay well.

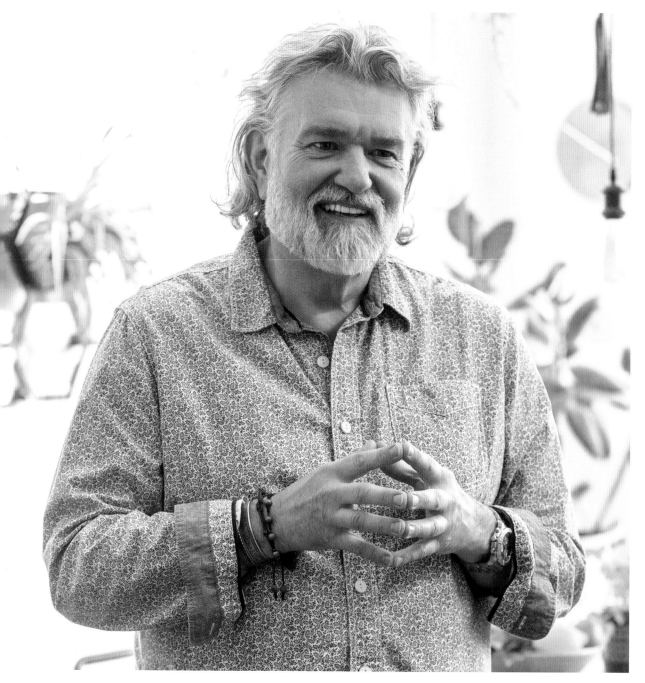

NUTRITIONAL INFO

While these recipes will help you control your weight, this is not a calorie-counting book as such, but we have included calorie counts, plus full nutritional details for your information. Unless otherwise noted, the figures are per serving, without any optional extras. Quantities are in grams. For salt, anything less than 0.1 grams of salt is listed as a trace.

CALORIES measure the amount of energy in the food. It can be tedious to count calories every day, but it's always useful to know the approximate number of calories in the food you eat to help your control your weight.

PROTEIN helps you feel satisfied, and we need protein to maintain our body's processes. Nuts and pulses, as well as meat, fish, eggs and dairy, are all good sources.

CARBOHYDRATES are made up of lots of sugar molecules bound together. Your digestion will turn them into sugar. But some are digested faster than others – and slowly digested carbs, like wholegrain foods, are better for your body because they produce less of a spike in your blood sugar. Many processed foods, such as ready meals, takeaways and sauces, contain added sugar. By avoiding processed foods, you'll benefit more than by worrying about different types of carbs.

SUGAR The figures listed are for the total amount of sugar in a dish, which includes the natural sugars in fruit, vegetables and dairy. It is the added sugar or free sugar, like the sugar added to hot drinks or used in puddings and cakes, that we need to limit and keep as low as possible for weight loss and good health.

FAT This figure is the total fat contained in a serving (monounsaturated, polyunsaturated and saturated). Monounsaturated fat – in foods such as nuts, seeds avocados and rapeseed and olive oil – and polyunsaturated fats in oily fish, nuts and seeds are better for you than saturated fat but they are all still high in calories. Fats are made up of strings of carbon atoms with lots of energy stored in the links in between them. Gram for gram, fat contains twice as many calories as protein or carbohydrate.

SATURATED FATS have different links between the carbon atoms (they are 'saturated' with hydrogen atoms). For good health we should aim to limit our intake of saturated fats, but we don't need to cut them out completely. It's recommended that less than 10 per cent of our total energy intake should come from saturated fats – about 22g a day for a women and 28g a day for men. The rest should come from mono and polyunsaturated fats

FIBRE remains largely undigested and so does not add many calories. It is contained in plant foods, such as fruit, vegetables, nuts and seeds, as well as in grains, and we need plenty of fibre in our diet to help digestion. Wholegrain bread, brown rice and brown pasta contain more fibre than refined varieties.

SALT The figures given are for the salt content in the ingredients, not any extra salt added to taste.

COOK'S NOTES

- Follow the recipes carefully so you don't change the calorie counts or nutritional details too much. Weigh your ingredients and use measuring spoons and a measuring jug.

- Use free-range eggs whenever possible. We generally use large eggs unless otherwise specified.

- Peel vegetables, onions and garlic unless otherwise specified. Sometimes we like to leave skins on where appropriate to increase the fibre content of a dish.

- We've given prep and cook times as a guide, but bear in mind that prep times don't include popping to the shop for an onion! We've made oven temperatures as accurate as possible, but ovens differ, so be prepared to cook your dish for a longer or shorter time if necessary.

FEED YOUR IMMUNITY

We need a strong immune system to protect us from infections, but did you know that about 70 per cent of our immune tissue is in our gut? Yes, gut health really is important, and we can nourish our gut – and our immune system – with good food. This means eating a wide range of vegetables, fruit and other unprocessed foods rich in vitamins and minerals, and we've learned there are some that are particularly worth including in our diet. These include leeks, onions, Jerusalem artichokes, squash, red peppers, shiitake mushrooms, nuts and seeds, wholegrain cereals and oily fish. Fermented foods, such as sauerkraut and kefir, are also excellent for boosting gut health and immunity.

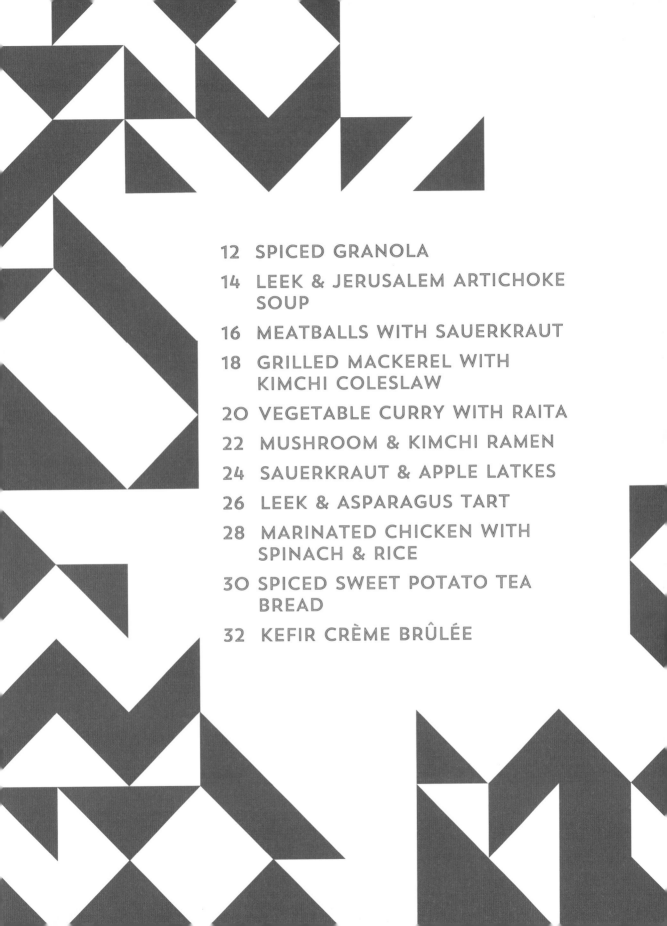

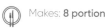
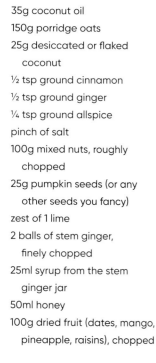

35g coconut oil

150g porridge oats

25g desiccated or flaked
  coconut

½ tsp ground cinnamon

½ tsp ground ginger

¼ tsp ground allspice

pinch of salt

100g mixed nuts, roughly
  chopped

25g pumpkin seeds (or any
  other seeds you fancy)

zest of 1 lime

2 balls of stem ginger,
  finely chopped

25ml syrup from the stem
  ginger jar

50ml honey

100g dried fruit (dates, mango,
  pineapple, raisins), chopped

SPICED GRANOLA

This is packed with immune-boosting ingredients like nuts and seeds and is a great nutritious breakfast. We used to bake our granola in the oven, but this frying-pan version is quick and easy – and saves you heating up the oven. Enjoy with some fresh fruit and yoghurt and it will keep you going all morning.

Melt the coconut oil in a large frying pan. Mix the porridge oats, coconut and spices together with a generous pinch of salt. Add them to the frying pan and stir constantly for a minute or so, until the ingredients are completely combined with the oil. Spread the mixture over the pan and leave it to toast for a couple of minutes, then give it a stir. Spread it again and stir, then repeat for about 10 minutes until the dry ingredients are giving off a lightly toasted aroma.

Add the mixed nuts, pumpkin seeds and lime zest and cook for another couple of minutes. Mix the stem ginger, syrup and honey together and pour this over the contents of the frying pan. Stir again until the mixture coats the dry ingredients – make sure none of the pieces of ginger clump together. Cook for another 5 minutes, stirring regularly, then add the dried fruit. Remove the pan from the heat.

Line a large baking tray with baking parchment and tip the granola on to the tray. Spread it out to cool and crisp. You can squeeze the mixture into clumps if you like or leave it loose. Store in an airtight container.

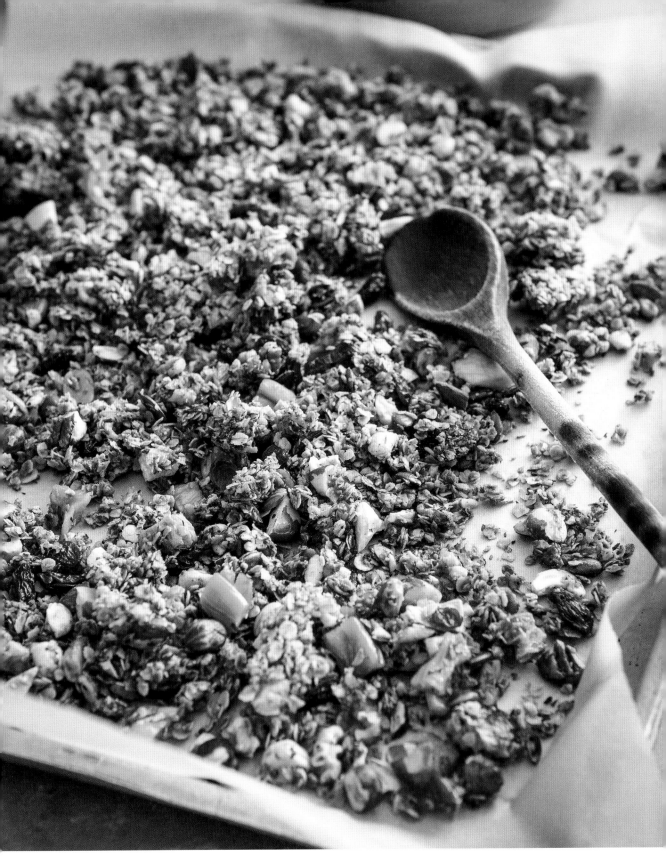

INFO PER SERVING: CALORIES 294 PROTEIN (G) 7 CARBS (G) 30 SUGAR (G) 18 FAT (G) 15 SATURATED FAT (G) 7 FIBRE (G) 3 SALT (G) 0.15

LEEK & JERUSALEM ARTICHOKE SOUP

1 tbsp olive oil

15g butter (or another 1 tbsp olive oil)

1 onion, finely chopped

1 celery stick, chopped

2 leeks, sliced

500g Jerusalem artichokes, scrubbed and chopped

1 tsp thyme leaves

2 garlic cloves, finely chopped

1 litre well-flavoured chicken or vegetable stock

salt and black pepper

To garnish

drizzle of olive or hazelnut oil

25g hazelnuts, toasted and lightly crushed

Jerusalem artichokes might make you windy but they are an excellent gut-friendly food and combined with leeks they make a super-tasty soup. They're a devil to peel though, so we're happy just to give them a good scrub and leave the peel on – means extra fibre too, so it's all good.

Heat the olive oil and butter, if using, in a large saucepan. Add the onion, celery, leeks and artichokes. Sauté over a high heat until the vegetables are starting to soften – this will take about 10 minutes.

Add the thyme leaves and garlic. Continue to cook for another couple of minutes, then season with salt and pepper. Pour in the stock, bring to the boil, then turn down the heat and simmer until the vegetables are completely tender – about another 15 minutes.

Blend the soup with either a stick or jug blender. If you like a completely smooth soup, pass it through a sieve as well, but it shouldn't be necessary.

Serve drizzled with oil and garnished with the hazelnuts.

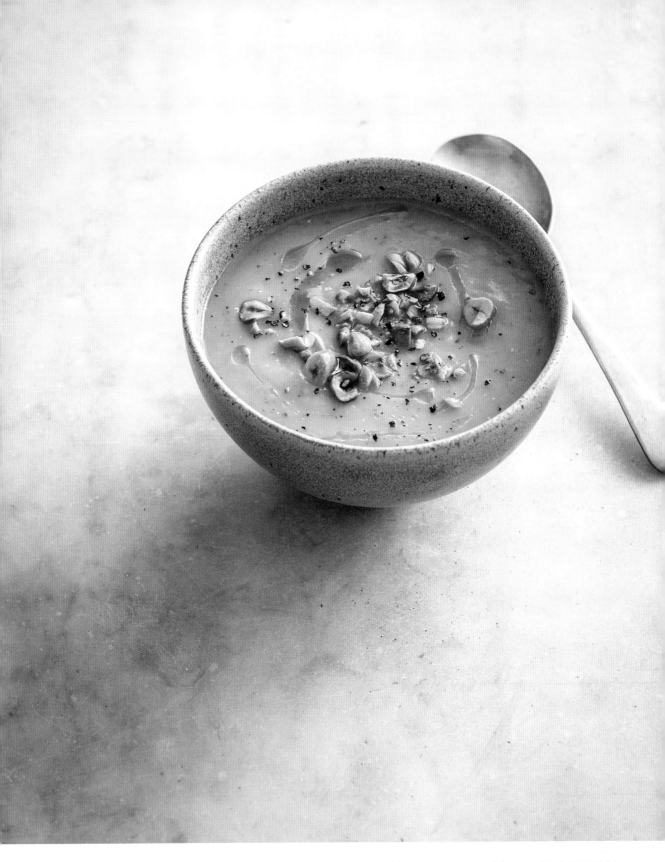

INFO PER SERVING: CALORIES 264 PROTEIN (G) 11 CARBS (G) 19 SUGAR (G) 7 FAT (G) 13.5 SATURATED FAT (G) 3 FIBRE (G) 10 SALT (G) 0.4

Meatballs

500g lean pork mince

1 apple, cored and coarsely grated

50g fresh breadcrumbs

1 tbsp wholegrain mustard

½ tsp dried sage, finely crumbled

salt and black pepper

Sauerkraut

1 tbsp olive oil

1 small onion, finely chopped

½ green pointed cabbage, finely shredded

2 garlic cloves, finely chopped

1 tsp juniper berries, lightly crushed

generous pinch of caraway seeds

300g sauerkraut (drained weight – shop-bought or see p.183)

2 tbsp tomato purée

To serve

new potatoes (optional)

MEATBALLS WITH SAUERKRAUT

This was inspired by those epic German dishes with sausage and sauerkraut. We're really into fermented foods and they're so good for your immune system. You can buy sauerkraut in the supermarket now or make your own from our recipe on page 183. It's perfect with these meatballs.

Preheat the oven to 200°C/Fan 180°C/Gas 6. Mix all the meatball ingredients in a bowl and season generously with salt and pepper. Divide the mixture into 16 balls and place them on a baking tray lined with baking paper. Bake in the oven for about 15 minutes until cooked through.

While the meatballs are cooking, heat the olive oil in a large sauté pan. Add the onion and cook for a few minutes over a high heat until it's starting to brown, then add the cabbage, garlic, juniper and caraway. Stir for a few more minutes until the cabbage collapses down but still looks fresh and green.

Taste the sauerkraut and rinse it briefly if it tastes too sour or vinegary, then add it to the pan. Dilute the tomato purée with 100ml of water and add it to the pan. Stir until everything is well combined.

Arrange the meatballs over the cabbage and sauerkraut. Cover and bring to the boil, then turn the heat down and simmer for 10 minutes to cook the tomato purée and blend the flavours. Serve on its own or with new potatoes, if you like.

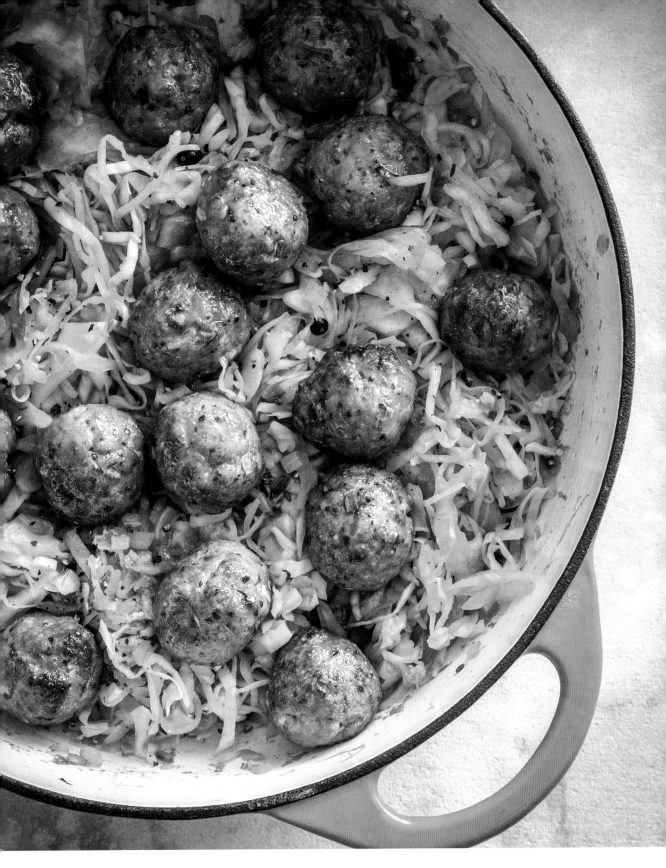

INFO PER SERVING: CALORIES 323 PROTEIN (G) 33 CARBS (G) 21 SUGAR (G) 12 FAT (G) 10 SATURATED FAT (G) 2.5 FIBRE (G) 9 SALT (G) 1.6

1 tbsp soy sauce

1 tsp sesame oil

10g root ginger, finely grated

4 mackerel fillets

1 tbsp olive oil

salt and black pepper

Kimchi coleslaw

½ green or white cabbage (about 300g), finely shredded

1 large carrot, coarsely grated or cut into matchsticks

4 spring onions, finely sliced

150g kimchi, finely chopped

1 tsp black or white sesame seeds

GRILLED MACKEREL WITH KIMCHI COLESLAW

Kimchi is another fermented food that's great for your gut, and adding some to coleslaw makes a really tasty mix that's just right with oily fish like mackerel. You can buy kimchi or make your own (see page 182). This makes a nice light lunch as it is or you could add some carbs, such as brown rice, for a heartier meal.

First make the coleslaw. Put the cabbage, carrot and spring onions in a colander and sprinkle with half a teaspoon of salt. Leave to stand for half an hour, tossing regularly, until the vegetables look slightly wet and collapsed. Drain, squeezing gently to get rid of any excess liquid, then stir through the kimchi.

For the mackerel, mix together the soy sauce, sesame oil and ginger. Season the fillets with salt and pepper, then dip each one, flesh-side down, in the soy mixture.

Heat the oil in a large frying pan. When it's hot, add the mackerel fillets, skin-side down, and fry them over a medium to high heat until the skin is crisp and pulls away easily from the pan. The flesh will have turned almost completely opaque. Carefully flip the fillets over, then cook for another minute.

Arrange the coleslaw over 4 plates and sprinkle with the sesame seeds. Top with the mackerel fillets and serve immediately.

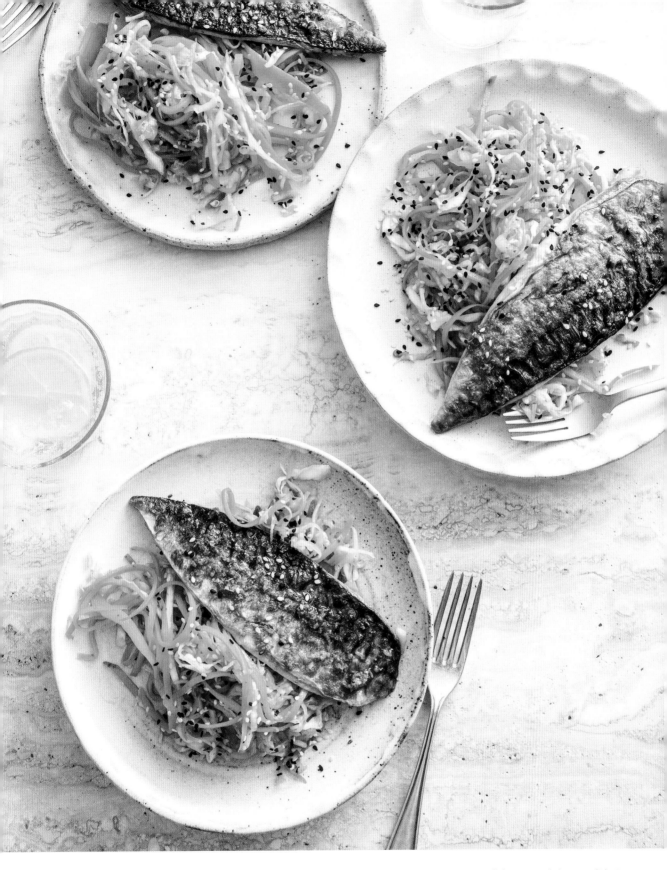

INFO PER SERVING: CALORIES 322 PROTEIN (G) 21 CARBS (G) 7 SUGAR (G) 6 FAT (G) 22.5 SATURATED FAT (G) 4.5 FIBRE (G) 5 SALT (G) 1.7

1 tbsp olive oil

a few curry leaves (optional)

1 large onion, sliced

400g new or salad potatoes, sliced

3 garlic cloves, finely chopped

15g root ginger, grated

1 tbsp curry powder

1 tbsp tamarind paste

400g cherry tomatoes

400g green beans, trimmed and halved

2 courgettes, sliced on the diagonal

squeeze of lemon or lime juice

salt and black pepper

Raita

250 live yoghurt or kefir

1 tsp chopped mint

To serve

a few mint leaves

a few coriander leaves

2 green chillies, finely sliced

VEGETABLE CURRY WITH RAITA

Everyone needs a good vegetable curry recipe and this light but surprisingly filling version really fits the bill. It helps you to reach your five a day target too. The curry leaves add a lovely smokiness to the flavour and balance well with the mint and coriander. Tamarind is rich in antioxidants, so is another good immune-boosting ingredient.

Heat the olive oil in a saucepan. Add the curry leaves, if using, and when they start crackling, add the onion and potatoes. Sauté over a medium heat until the onion has softened, while stirring regularly.

Add the garlic and ginger and cook for another couple of minutes, then stir in the curry powder, followed by the tamarind paste. Season with salt and pepper. Pour over 300ml of water and bring to the boil, then turn down the heat and partially cover the pan. Simmer for about 10 minutes.

Stir in the cherry tomatoes, then put the green beans and courgettes on top. Cover the pan again and leave to steam until the beans and courgettes are tender. Stir everything together, then taste and add a squeeze of lemon or lime juice.

To make the raita, mix the yoghurt or kefir with the mint and a generous pinch of salt. Serve the curry garnished with the herbs, with the green chillies and raita on the side.

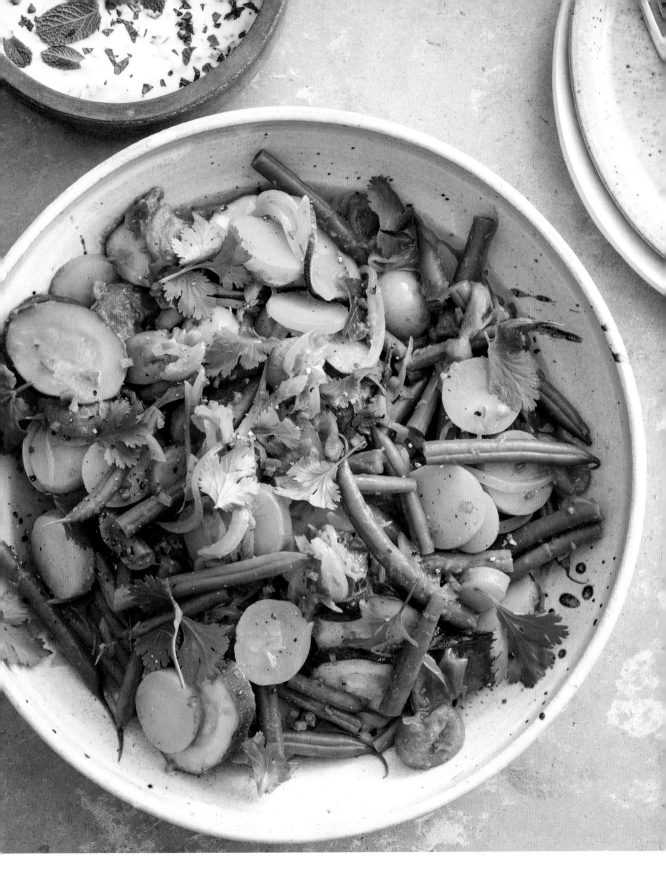

INFO PER SERVING: CALORIES 247   PROTEIN (G) 9   CARBS (G) 33   SUGAR (G) 14   FAT (G) 7   SATURATED FAT (G) 2   FIBRE (G) 10   SALT (G) 0.2

15g dried shiitake mushrooms

2 tbsp white miso paste

1.5 litres vegetable stock

15g root ginger, cut into
matchsticks

3 garlic cloves, finely sliced

2 tbsp soy sauce

250g fresh shiitake mushrooms,
sliced

250g pak choi or similar

250g chopped kimchi,
including the juice (shop-
bought or see p.182)

salt

To serve

4 nests of noodles

small bunch of coriander,
finely chopped

leaves from a small bunch
of mint, roughly chopped

drizzle of sesame or chilli oil

MUSHROOM & KIMCHI RAMEN

This is a really simple ramen that's easy to make and you don't have to strain the broth before adding the vegetables. Shiitake mushrooms are full of flavour and also provide phytochemicals, which are believed to help boost immunity. Adding the kimchi just before serving preserves its nutritional qualities.

First make the broth. Crumble the dried mushrooms into a large saucepan. Whisk the miso with some of the stock to loosen it, then when you have a smooth, pourable liquid, add this to the saucepan along with the remaining stock, the ginger and garlic. Season with salt and bring to the boil, then simmer for 10 minutes.

Add the soy sauce, fresh shiitake and pak choi. Simmer until the vegetables are cooked through, then stir in the kimchi. Remove the pan from the heat.

Cook the noodles according to the packet instructions and divide them between 4 large bowls. Ladle over the broth and vegetables, then sprinkle with the herbs. Drizzle with sesame or chilli oil before serving.

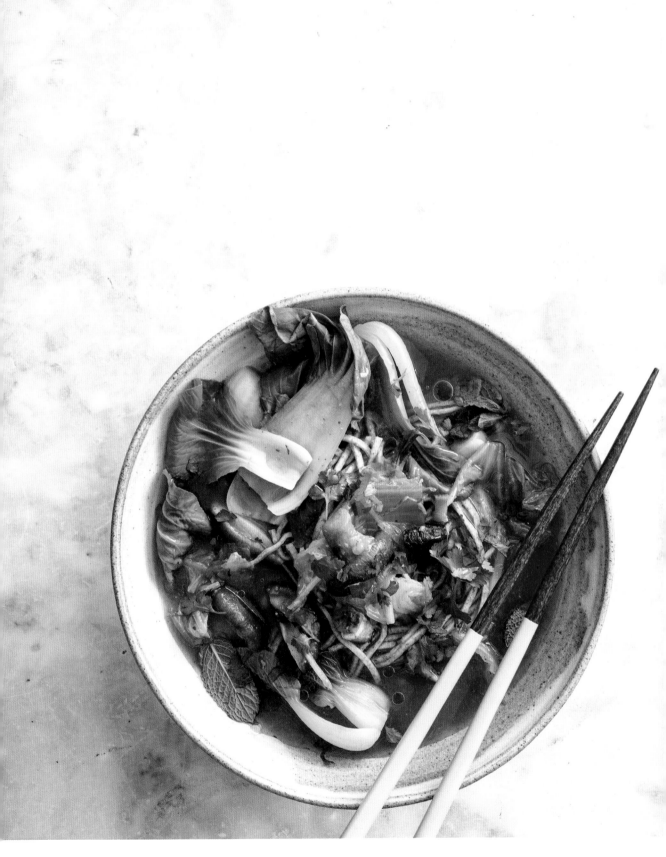

INFO PER SERVING: CALORIES 88   PROTEIN (G) 6   CARBS (G) 10   SUGAR (G) 5.5   FAT (G) 2   SATURATED FAT (G) 1   FIBRE (G) 4   SALT (G) 3.5

Serves: **4** Prep: **10 minutes + standing** Cooking time: **about 15 minutes**

300g floury potatoes, coarsely
grated
1 large carrot, coarsely grated
1 small onion, finely chopped
1 small eating apple, cored
and grated
100g sauerkraut, drained
and roughly chopped
(shop-bought or see p.183)
2 tbsp olive oil
salt and black pepper

To serve
200ml thick kefir or soured
cream
a few dill fronds, finely
chopped
½ tsp garlic powder
zest of ½ lemon
squeeze of lemon juice

SAUERKRAUT & APPLE LATKES

Everyone loves latkes and making them with some sauerkraut as
well as apple makes them healthier and better for you. There's no
flour or matzo meal in these either, so they are gluten-free. Nice
served with the kefir or soured cream or you could add poached
eggs and/or grilled tomatoes.

Put the potatoes, carrot, onion and apple in a colander and sprinkle with half a
teaspoon of salt. Leave to stand for half an hour, then squeeze out as much liquid
as you can with your hands. Pile everything on to a clean tea towel and add the
sauerkraut. Twist the tea towel into a bundle and squeeze again, extracting as
much liquid as possible.

Transfer to a bowl and season with pepper, then divide the mixture into 8. Heat
a tablespoon of the olive oil in a large frying pan. Squeeze the mixture tightly into
rounds and place half of them into the frying pan, pressing them down firmly. Fry for
3–4 minutes on each side until crisp and golden brown, then place them on a plate
lined with kitchen paper to drain. Repeat with the remaining oil and latkes mixture.

To make the sauce, put the kefir or soured cream in a bowl and whisk in the dill,
garlic powder, lemon zest and juice. Season with salt and black pepper. Serve
the latkes with the sauce.

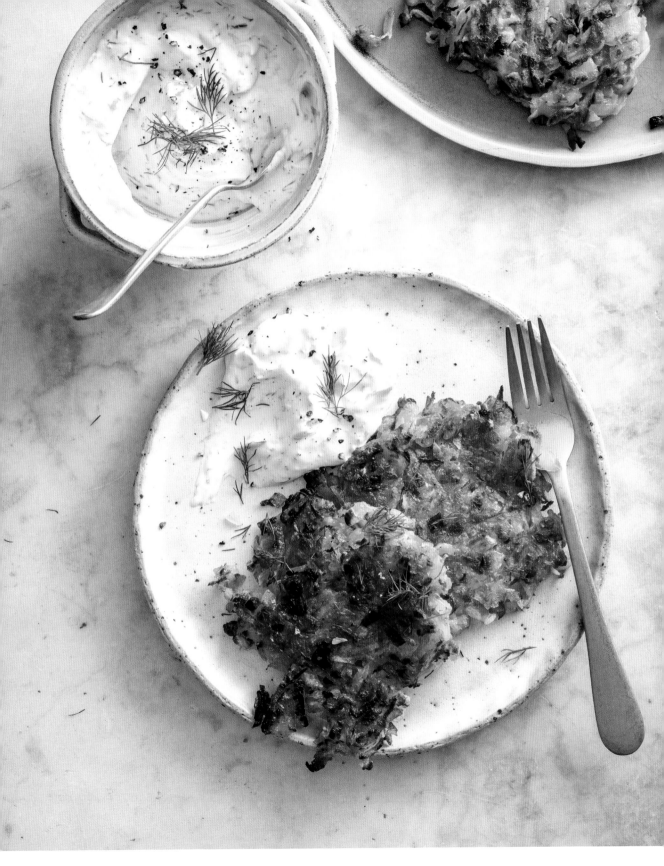

INFO PER SERVING: CALORIES 182 PROTEIN (G) 4 CARBS (G) 23 SUGAR (G) 9 FAT (G) 7.5 SATURATED FAT (G) 2 FIBRE (G) 4 SALT (G) 0.5

LEEK & ASPARAGUS TART

Base

250g strong white flour (or half white, half wholemeal), plus extra for dusting

½ tsp salt

½ tsp fast-action dried yeast

1 tbsp olive oil

150ml tepid water

Topping

1 tbsp olive oil

1 tbsp butter

500g leeks, finely sliced

1 thyme sprig, left whole

leaves from 1 tarragon sprig, finely chopped

2 garlic cloves, finely chopped

100g asparagus tips

50ml crème fraiche

1 egg

100g mature Cheddar or Gruyère, grated

1 tsp Dijon mustard

salt and black pepper

Asparagus contains prebiotic fibre that boosts friendly bacteria in the gut. It partners well with leeks to top our version of the Flemish leek tart known as flamiche. Quite a bit of cheese in this, but we've used a bread-style base instead of pastry, so the dish is not too high in fat.

First make the dough. Put the flour in a bowl and mix in the salt before adding the yeast. Drizzle in the olive oil, then work in the tepid water to make a sticky dough. Leave it to stand for 10 minutes, then turn it out on to a floured surface and knead until soft and elastic. Put the dough back in the bowl, cover it with a damp tea towel and leave until the dough has doubled in size.

For the topping, put the oil and butter in a large, lidded sauté pan. Add the leeks, along with the thyme, tarragon and garlic, then season with salt and pepper. Stir to combine, then cover the pan and leave the leeks to sweat over a low heat. Keep stirring at intervals to make sure the leeks aren't catching on the base of the pan.

After about 8 minutes, lay the asparagus tips on top. Cook for a further 2 minutes, then remove from the heat and leave to cool. Remove the asparagus from the pan and set aside. Take out the thyme sprig.

Beat the crème fraiche and egg together. Season with salt and pepper, then stir in the leeks and 75g of the cheese.

Preheat the oven to 200°C/Fan 180°C/Gas 6. Take a baking tin measuring about 25 x 35cm. Press the dough into the tin, making sure it has a slightly raised rim all the way around it. Spread the mustard over the dough, then top with the leek mixture. Arrange the asparagus tips over the leeks, then sprinkle the remaining cheese on top.

Bake in the preheated oven for about 25 minutes until the base is crisp and golden and the topping is lightly browned in places. Serve hot or at room temperature.

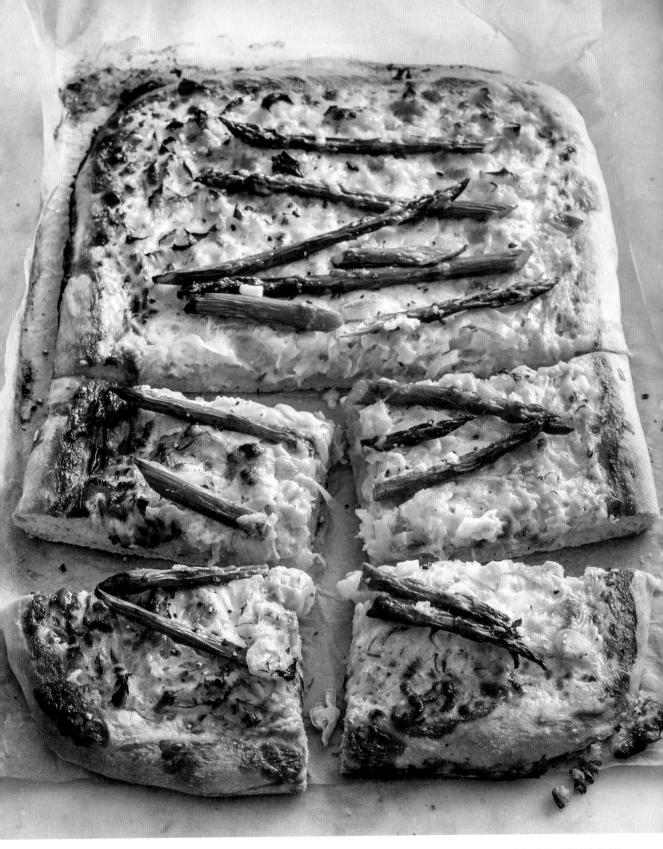

INFO PER 4 SERVINGS/6 SERVINGS: CALORIES 552/348   PROTEIN (G) 19/13   CARBS (G) 52/34   SUGAR (G) 4/2.5   FAT (G) 25/17

SATURATED FAT (G) 12/8   FIBRE (G) 6/4   SALT (G) 1.3/0.9

8 chicken thigh fillets or
    8 drumsticks, skinned

Marinade

200g yoghurt or kefir

1 tbsp tahini

pinch of saffron, lightly crushed

3 garlic cloves, crushed

2 tbsp finely chopped
    coriander

2 tsp baharat powder

juice and zest of 1 lemon

salt and black pepper

To serve

100g baby spinach, washed

250g cooked brown rice
    (100g uncooked weight)

3 spring onions, finely chopped

1 tbsp olive oil

juice of ½ lemon

seeds from a small
    pomegranate

leaves from a few coriander
    sprigs

leaves from a few mint sprigs

25g pumpkin seeds

lemon wedges

MARINATED CHICKEN WITH SPINACH & RICE

Just remember to marinate your chicken and this is a doddle to make and is packed with goodness. Apparently, rice that has been cooked and then cooled has improved health benefits: the starch in the rice becomes resistant starch – a sort of fibre that's good for your gut. Pomegranates are a good source of dietary fibre, vitamins C and K and folate.

Cut slashes in the chicken flesh, going right through to the bone if using drumsticks. Mix all the marinade ingredients together in a bowl and season with salt and pepper. Add the chicken, rubbing the marinade into all the cuts. Cover and leave in the fridge until you are ready to cook – preferably for at least an hour or overnight if necessary.

When you are ready to cook the chicken, heat a griddle pan until it's too hot to hold your hand over. Scrape off any excess marinade from the chicken pieces, then grill them on all sides until cooked through and well charred. The drumsticks will take up to 20 minutes, the thighs up to 15.

Toss the spinach with the cooked rice and spring onions, then dress with the olive oil and lemon juice. Sprinkle over the pomegranate seeds, herbs and pumpkin seeds. Serve with the chicken and some lemon wedges.

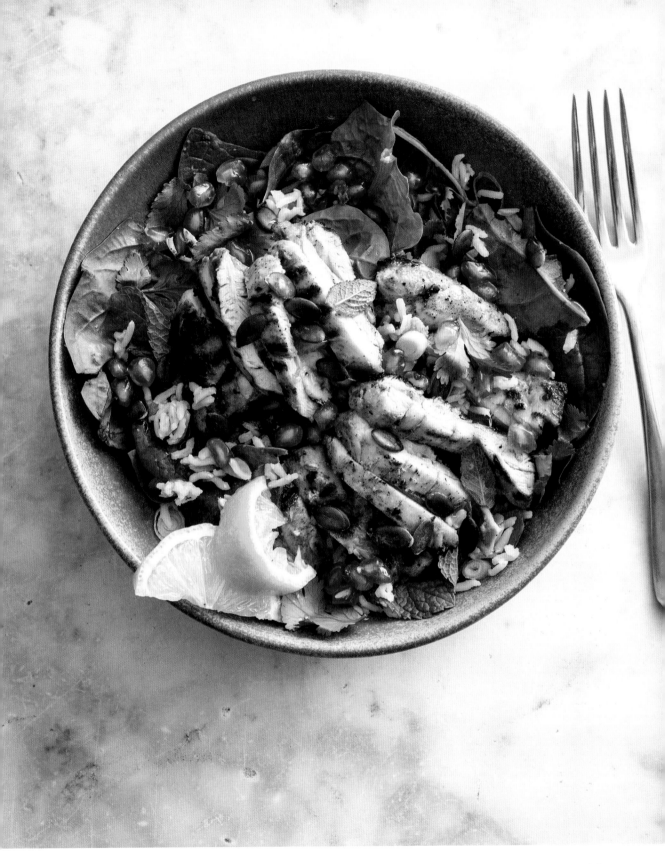

INFO PER SERVING: CALORIES 431   PROTEIN (G) 49   CARBS (G) 22   SUGAR (G) 4   FAT (G) 16   SATURATED FAT (G) 4   FIBRE (G) 2.5   SALT (G) 0.5

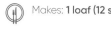
1 sweet potato (about 350g)

300g plain flour (wholemeal or white)

1 tbsp baking powder

1 tsp ground cinnamon

1 tsp mixed spice

100g light brown soft sugar

pinch of salt

100g dates, finely diced

3 eggs

75–100ml milk

SPICED SWEET POTATO TEA BREAD

If you're making the stuffed sweet potatoes on page 56, pop an extra one in the oven and then bake this spicy tea bread for an afternoon treat with your cuppa. Otherwise, you could steam the sweet potato. Delicious toasted and buttered.

Preheat the oven to 200°C/Fan 180°C/Gas 6. Pierce the sweet potato all over with a skewer and put it in the oven for 45–50 minutes until tender. Remove from the oven and peel when it's cool enough to handle. Mash, then leave to cool completely.

Reduce the oven temperature to 170°C/Fan 150°C/Gas 3½ and line a 900g loaf tin with baking parchment.

Put the flour, baking powder, spices and sugar in a large bowl. Add a pinch of salt and mix thoroughly. Add the dates, making sure they are well coated with the flour.

Beat the eggs into the mashed sweet potato, then fold this mixture into the dry ingredients. Add just enough milk to make a reluctant dropping consistency.

Scrape the mixture into the prepared tin, then bake for 55–60 minutes until the loaf is well risen, springy to the touch and has slightly shrunk away from the sides.

Turn out the loaf out and leave to cool, then wrap and store in an airtight tin. It will have a better texture after a couple of days.

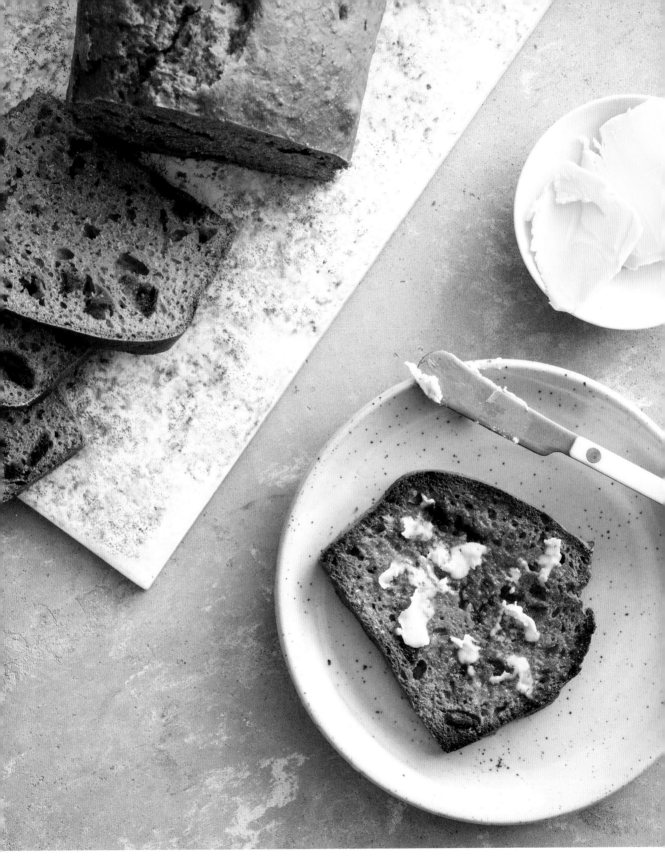

INFO PER SLICE: CALORIES 190   PROTEIN (G) 5   CARBS (G) 36   SUGAR (G) 12.5   FAT (G) 2   SATURATED FAT (G) 1   FIBRE (G) 2   SALT (G) 0.5

1 large or 2 small ripe mangoes, peeled and sliced

zest of 1 lime

¼ tsp ground cinnamon

¼ tsp ground ginger

1 tbsp runny honey

125g crème fraiche

125g thick kefir (shop-bought or see p.181)

4 tsp granulated sugar

KEFIR CRÈME BRÛLÉE

You might think that finding a reasonably healthy crème brûlée recipe is like the search for the holy grail, but we think we've done it. Yes, this is usually a really indulgent dessert but our recipe using kefir and no eggs is – almost – guilt-free and ridiculously simple! Kefir is a probiotic, so contains live bacteria that are good for your gut and your immune system. Epic!

Toss the mango slices with the lime zest, cinnamon and ginger. Divide the slices between 4 ramekin dishes.

Put the honey in a bowl and gradually incorporate the crème fraiche until smooth, then fold in the kefir. Spoon this mixture over the mango slices in each ramekin and smooth over the tops. Cover and put in the fridge to chill and thicken.

Just before you are ready to serve, preheat the grill. Sprinkle each crème brûlée with a teaspoon of sugar and place under the grill until the sugar has melted and browned. Carefully remove the ramekins from the grill – the topping should harden very quickly. Serve immediately.

 Tip: If you have a blow torch, you could use that instead of the grill for browning the brûlée tops.

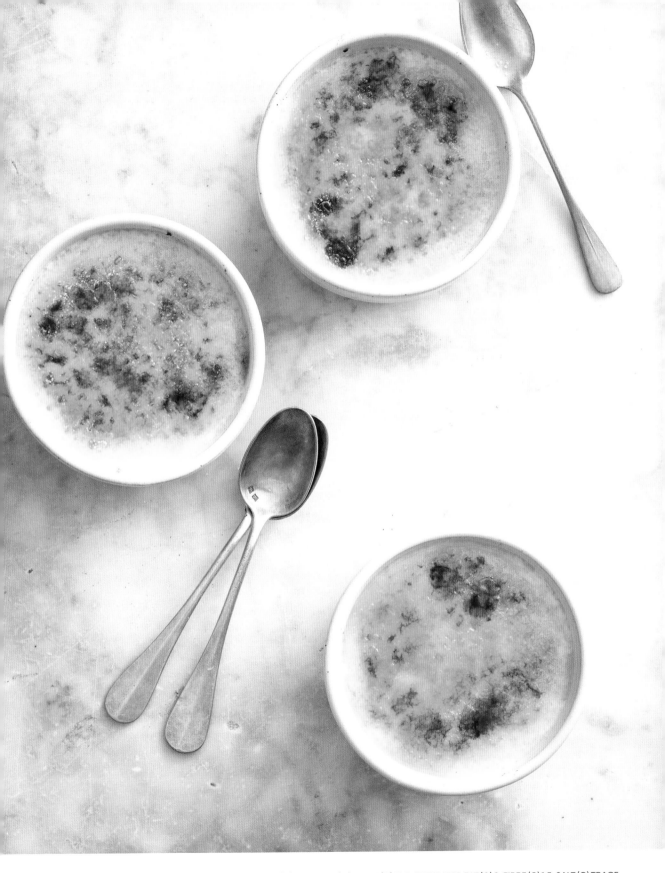

INFO PER SERVING: CALORIES 202 PROTEIN (G) 2 CARBS (G) 17 SUGAR (G) 17 FAT (G) 13.5 SATURATED FAT (G) 9 FIBRE (G) 1.5 SALT (G) TRACE

EATING FOR ENERGY

We need food to fuel our bodies and give us the energy to get through the day, so that means choosing good carbs combined with protein, fruit and veg and healthy fats. Simple carbohydrates, such as cakes and sweets, might give you a quick boost, but you'll soon crash, while whole grains, oats, beans and pulses are slow-release carbs and so help you maintain energy levels throughout the day. Other foods that are important for energy are dark-green leafy veg, red meat and poultry, which provide B vitamins and iron. And don't forget to drink water – good hydration helps keep up energy levels.

8 lamb kidneys

1 tbsp olive oil

1 shallot, finely sliced

2 garlic cloves, finely chopped

50ml dry sherry

100ml chicken stock

1 tbsp tomato purée

2 tsp Dijon mustard

1 tsp smoked paprika

½ tsp hot paprika or cayenne

dash of Worcestershire sauce

squeeze of lemon juice

small bunch of parsley, finely
    chopped

To serve

buttered toast

DEVILLED KIDNEYS

If you're a fan of kidneys, this is the best breakfast ever. It's an old-fashioned classic and deserves to be on our tables at any time of day. Kidneys are an excellent source of B vitamins, which are essential for the release of energy from food.

First prepare the kidneys. Cut them in half and cut out the white cores – be sure to do this carefully, as bits of core can spoil the dish. Cut each kidney in half again so they are quartered.

Heat the olive oil in a large frying pan. Add the shallot and fry it over a medium-high heat until softened and lightly browned, then add the garlic and cook for a few more moments. Push the shallot and garlic to one side and turn up the heat. Add the kidneys and fry for a couple of minutes just to sear. Pour in the sherry and leave it to bubble and reduce.

Whisk the stock with the tomato purée, mustard, paprika and hot paprika or cayenne. Pour this over the kidneys and add a good dash of Worcestershire sauce. Bring to the boil again and leave to simmer, stirring regularly, for 3–4 minutes until the sauce has reduced down and thickened. Squeeze over some lemon juice and sprinkle with chopped parsley.

Serve on hot buttered toast or folded into flatbreads.

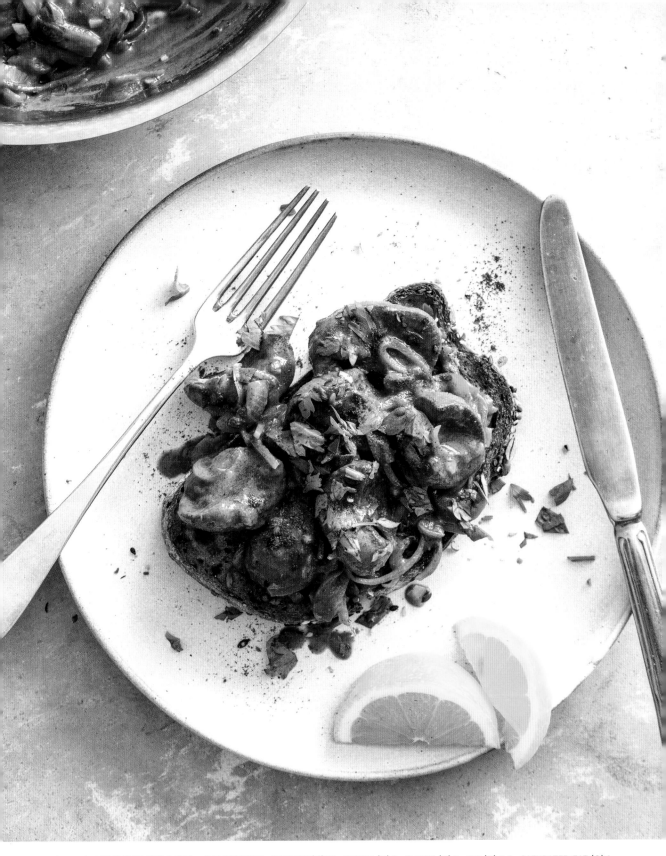

INFO PER SERVING (KIDNEYS ONLY):   CALORIES 110   PROTEIN (G) 12   CARBS (G) 1   SUGAR (G) 1   FAT (G) 4.5   SATURATED FAT (G) 1

FIBRE (G) 0.5   SALT (G) 0.5

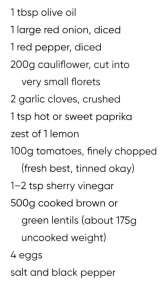

1 tbsp olive oil

1 large red onion, diced

1 red pepper, diced

200g cauliflower, cut into
very small florets

2 garlic cloves, crushed

1 tsp hot or sweet paprika

zest of 1 lemon

100g tomatoes, finely chopped
(fresh best, tinned okay)

1–2 tsp sherry vinegar

500g cooked brown or
green lentils (about 175g
uncooked weight)

4 eggs

salt and black pepper

To serve

a few parsley sprigs,
finely chopped

lemon wedges

live yoghurt or kefir (optional)

BRAISED LENTILS & EGGS

Lentils are great energy-boosters because they provide slow-release carbs and this dish is also packed with delicious veg. Good served with a simple green salad for lunch or a light supper, or with toast for breakfast or brunch to set you up for the day.

Heat the olive oil in a large, lidded sauté pan. Add the red onion, red pepper and cauliflower florets. Sauté over a high heat, stirring regularly, for about 5 minutes until the veg are starting to brown, then add a splash of water, cover and turn down the heat. Leave to cook for a further 5 minutes or until the vegetables are cooked but still have a little bite to them.

Add the garlic, paprika and lemon zest. Stir for another minute or so, then stir in the tomatoes and 1 teaspoon of sherry vinegar. Stir in the cooked lentils and 300ml of water, then season with salt and pepper.

Bring to the boil and simmer for 5 minutes just to combine the flavours. Taste and add the remaining sherry vinegar if you like. Make 4 wells in the lentils and crack in the eggs. Season the eggs, cover the pan and simmer until the egg whites are just set – another 5–8 minutes.

Sprinkle with parsley and serve with lemon wedges and some dollops of live yoghurt or kefir, if using.

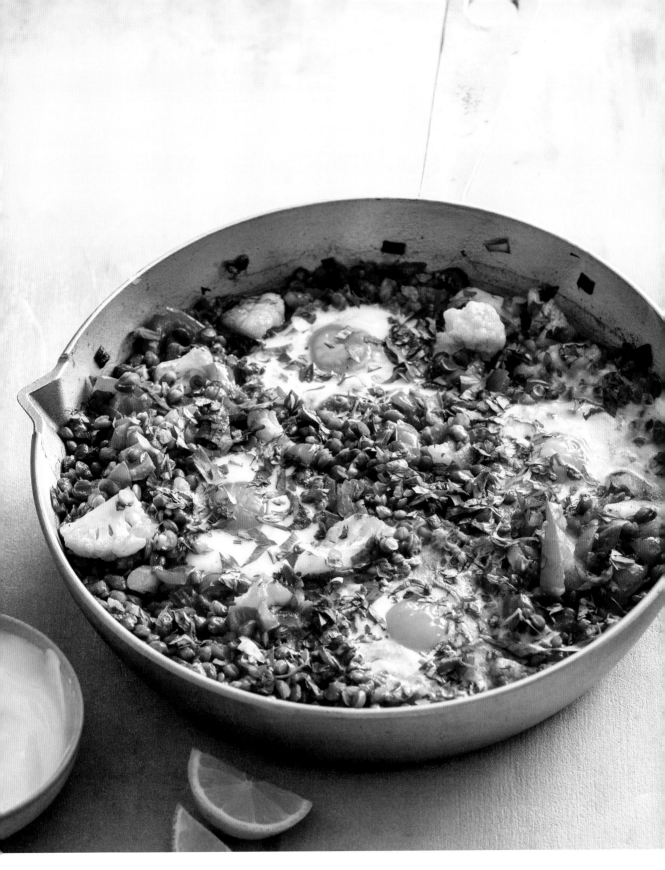

INFO PER SERVING: CALORIES 300 PROTEIN (G) 21 CARBS (G) 28 SUGAR (G) 7 FAT (G) 10 SATURATED FAT (G) 2 FIBRE (G) 9.5 SALT (G) 0.3

2 tbsp olive oil

1 onion, finely chopped

1 celery stick, finely diced

100g squash or pumpkin, peeled and finely diced

1 large courgette, coarsely grated

2 garlic cloves, finely chopped

1 tsp dried oregano or mixed Italian herbs

zest of 1 lemon

100g frozen spinach, defrosted

100g frozen peas (no need to defrost)

250g short pasta (such as fusilli)

up to 700ml vegetable stock

100g ricotta or similar cream cheese (soft goat's cheese is very good)

a few basil leaves, shredded

salt and black pepper

To serve (optional)

squeeze of lemon juice

vegetarian Parmesan-style cheese, grated

VEGGIE PASTA WITH RICOTTA

Pasta is always good for a boost, particularly if you use a wholewheat version and cook it al dente because it releases energy more slowly. And cooking the pasta by this absorption method means that it takes up all the flavours and no nutrients are wasted. Nice selection of veggies here – so this is good for getting your five a day – but feel free to vary them as you like.

Heat the oil in a large saucepan. Add the onion, celery, squash and courgette. Cook over a low to medium heat for several minutes, stirring regularly, until the courgette has collapsed down and reduced in volume and the onion has started to soften. Add the garlic and cook for a further couple of minutes.

Add the oregano, lemon zest, spinach, peas and pasta to the pan and season generously with salt and pepper. Pour over just enough stock to cover – the amount will vary depending on what type of pasta you use, but you'll probably need just over 600ml. Stir again and press the pasta down into the stock. Cover the pan and bring to the boil.

Turn the heat down so the pasta is cooking at just below boiling point – you don't want a fast boil here but something a bit faster than a simmer. Cook for about 12 minutes until the pasta is al dente and most of the liquid has been absorbed. Remove the pan from the heat and leave to stand for a further 5 minutes.

Stir in the ricotta or cream cheese along with the basil. When the cheese has melted, taste and add a squeeze of lemon juice if you like. Serve in shallow bowls with more black pepper and grated cheese, if using.

 Tip: You could use shredded kale instead of spinach, which should be added at the same time as the courgette.

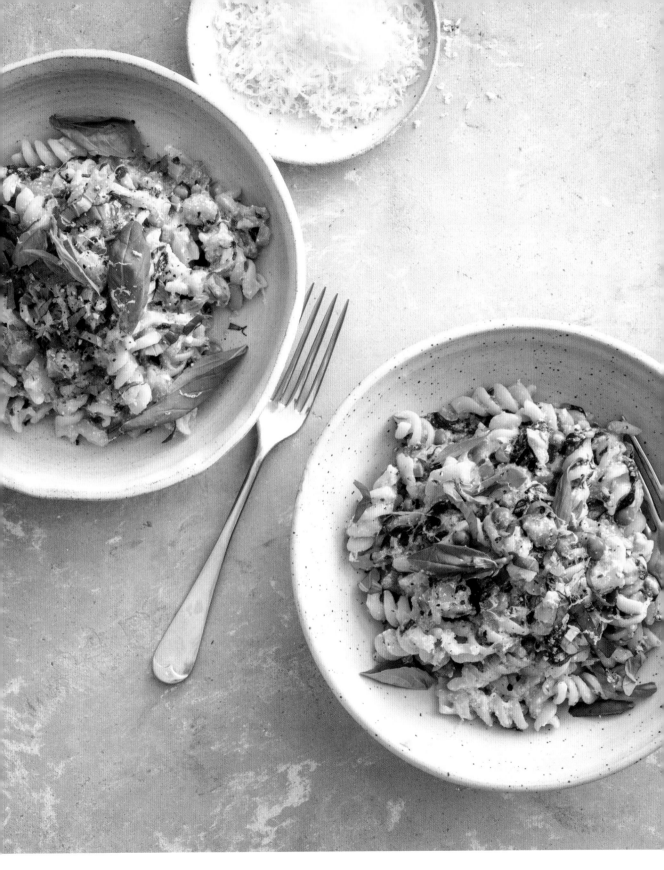

INFO PER SERVING: CALORIES 390 PROTEIN (G) 14.5 CARBS (G) 55.5 SUGAR (G) 8 FAT (G) 11 SATURATED FAT (G) 3 FIBRE (G) 7.5 SALT (G) 0.26

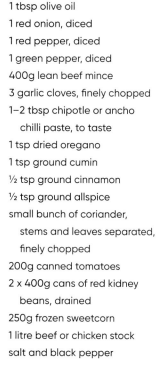

1 tbsp olive oil

1 red onion, diced

1 red pepper, diced

1 green pepper, diced

400g lean beef mince

3 garlic cloves, finely chopped

1–2 tbsp chipotle or ancho
 chilli paste, to taste

1 tsp dried oregano

1 tsp ground cumin

½ tsp ground cinnamon

½ tsp ground allspice

small bunch of coriander,
 stems and leaves separated,
 finely chopped

200g canned tomatoes

2 x 400g cans of red kidney
 beans, drained

250g frozen sweetcorn

1 litre beef or chicken stock

salt and black pepper

To garnish

100g tortilla chips

75g Cheddar, grated (optional)

To serve

pickled jalapeños (optional)

CHUNKY BEEF CHILLI SOUP

A real winter warmer, this soup contains beef and red kidney beans for energy and plenty of healthy spices. Nourishing and super tasty, it will keep you going for hours – it's worth making a big batch and stashing some in the freezer for another time. If you've made our fajitas spice mix on page 185, you can use a tablespoon of that instead of the individual spices listed.

Heat the olive oil in a large saucepan. Add the onion and peppers and sauté over a low to medium heat until the onion has started to soften and turn translucent. Turn up the heat and add the beef mince. Cook until well browned, then stir in the garlic and cook for a further minute.

Stir in the chipotle or chilli paste, the spices and coriander stems, followed by the tomatoes, beans and sweetcorn. Pour in the stock, then season with salt and pepper and bring to the boil. Partially cover the pan with a lid, turn down the heat and simmer for 20 minutes.

Serve the soup in bowls, add the tortilla chips and sprinkle with cheese, if using. Alternatively, spread the tortilla chips over a baking tray, sprinkle them with the cheese and put under a hot grill for a few minutes before adding them to the soup. Sprinkle with the jalapeños and coriander leaves before serving.

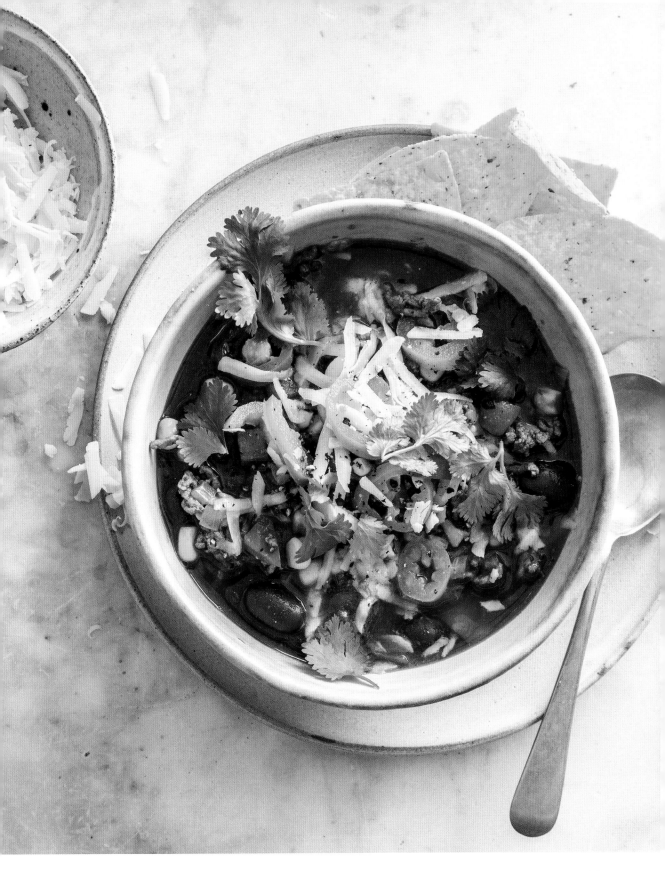

INFO PER SERVING: CALORIES 615 PROTEIN (G) 47 CARBS (G) 48 SUGAR (G) 12 FAT (G) 22 SATURATED FAT (G) 6 FIBRE (G) 18 SALT (G) 1.4

VEGGIE TACOS

1 red onion, finely sliced

½ tsp sea salt

1½ limes

1 tbsp olive oil

2 garlic cloves, finely chopped

1 tsp chilli paste

generous pinch of cinnamon

1 tsp dried oregano

200g cavolo nero, shredded

400g can of black, red kidney
   or pinto beans, drained

200g cherry tomatoes, halved
   or quartered

salt and black pepper

Sauce

zest of 1 lime

juice of 2 limes

1 avocado, stoned, peeled
   and mashed

a small bunch of coriander,
   roughly chopped

100ml live yoghurt or kefir

To serve

8 small corn tortillas, warmed

100g feta cheese, crumbled
   (optional)

2 tbsp pumpkin seeds

a few coriander sprigs

pickled jalapeños (optional)

Like other pulses, black beans are an excellent source of protein and are also high in fibre. We're often advised to 'eat the rainbow' in terms of veg and the selection here fits the bill.

Put the red onion in a bowl and add half a teaspoon of sea salt. Add the juice of 1 lime and toss, then set aside for at least half an hour.

For the sauce, put the lime zest and juice in a food processor with the avocado and coriander. Season with salt and pepper and process until the coriander has broken down. Add the yoghurt or kefir and blend again until you have a pale green sauce flecked with coriander. If the sauce is too thick to drizzle, thin it out with a little water.

Heat the olive oil in a sauté pan. Add the garlic and cook for a minute, then stir in the chilli paste, cinnamon and oregano. Add 100ml of water and the cavolo nero, then season with salt and pepper. Stir until the cavolo nero starts to collapse down, then cover the pan with a lid and leave to braise over a low heat for a few minutes until the cavolo is cooked through. Add the beans to warm through and squeeze over the juice of half a lime. Remove the pan from the heat and add the tomatoes.

Pile the bean mixture in the middle of the warm tortillas. Sprinkle over some feta, if using, add the pumpkin seeds and the drained red onion, then drizzle with the sauce. Garnish with coriander and pickled jalapeños, if using.

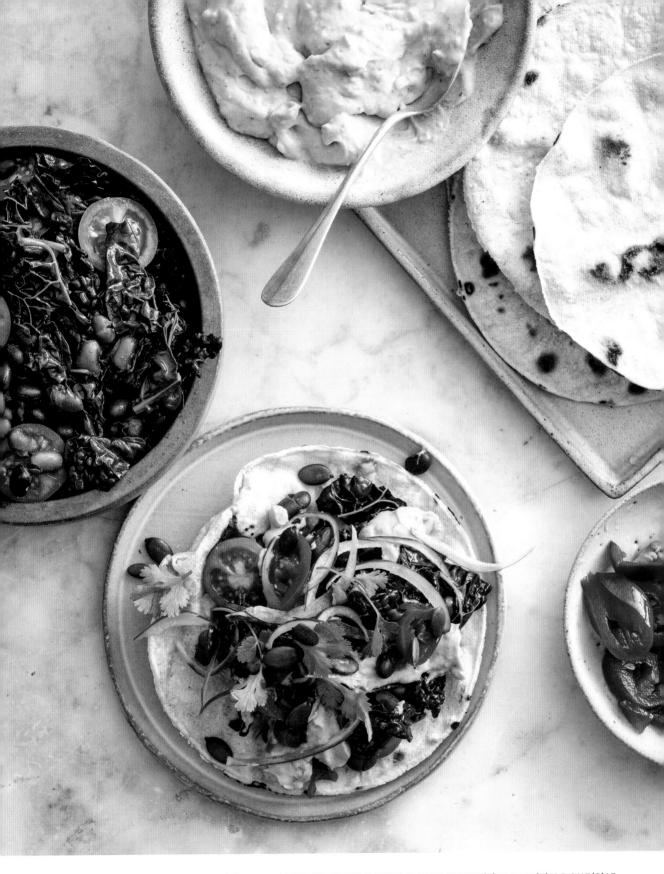

INFO PER SERVING: CALORIES 345 PROTEIN (G) 22 CARBS (G) 75 SUGAR (G) 8.5 FAT (G) 26 SATURATED FAT (G) 7.5 FIBRE (G) 10.5 SALT (G) 1.7

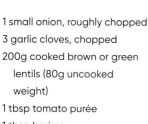

1 small onion, roughly chopped

3 garlic cloves, chopped

200g cooked brown or green lentils (80g uncooked weight)

1 tbsp tomato purée

1 tbsp harissa

300g minced lamb

1 tsp dried mint

salt and black pepper

Dressing

large pinch of saffron

large pinch of sea salt

1 tbsp tahini

½ tsp honey

juice of ½ lemon

200ml thick yoghurt or kefir

1 small garlic clove, crushed

Wholemeal couscous

150g wholemeal couscous

1 tbsp olive oil

juice of 1 orange

150ml warm water

1 small red onion, finely chopped

2 tomatoes, finely chopped

1 small bunch of parsley, finely chopped

1 small bunch of mint, finely chopped

LAMB KOFTA WITH TAHINI DRESSING & COUSCOUS

There's everything you need in this tasty recipe – juicy protein-rich kofta, flavoursome fibre with the couscous, all drizzled with a tahini and kefir dressing. Super healthy and super delicious, this is a real keeper we reckon. You'll need eight skewers, soaked for half an hour if they're made from bamboo.

To make the kofta, put the onion and garlic into a food processor and blend until very finely chopped. Add all the remaining kofta ingredients and season with salt and pepper. Continue to process until everything is well combined. Chill for half an hour. Divide the mixture into 8 pieces and mould around the skewers.

While the kofta mixture is chilling, make the dressing. Put the saffron in a bowl with a large pinch of sea salt and crush with a pestle or the back of a wooden spoon. Add the tahini, honey and lemon juice and whisk to combine. Stir in the yoghurt or kefir and the garlic.

Put the couscous in a bowl with a generous pinch of salt, the olive oil and the orange juice. Pour over the warm water, then cover and leave to stand until all the liquid has been absorbed. Fluff up with a fork, then stir in the onion, tomato and herbs.

To cook the kofta, heat a grill or griddle pan until very hot and arrange the skewers over it. Grill for a few minutes on each side until just cooked through with char lines. If you prefer, you could bake the kofta in a preheated oven (200°C/Fan 180°C/Gas 6) for 15 minutes.

Serve the couscous and the kofta with the dressing drizzled over the top.

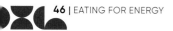

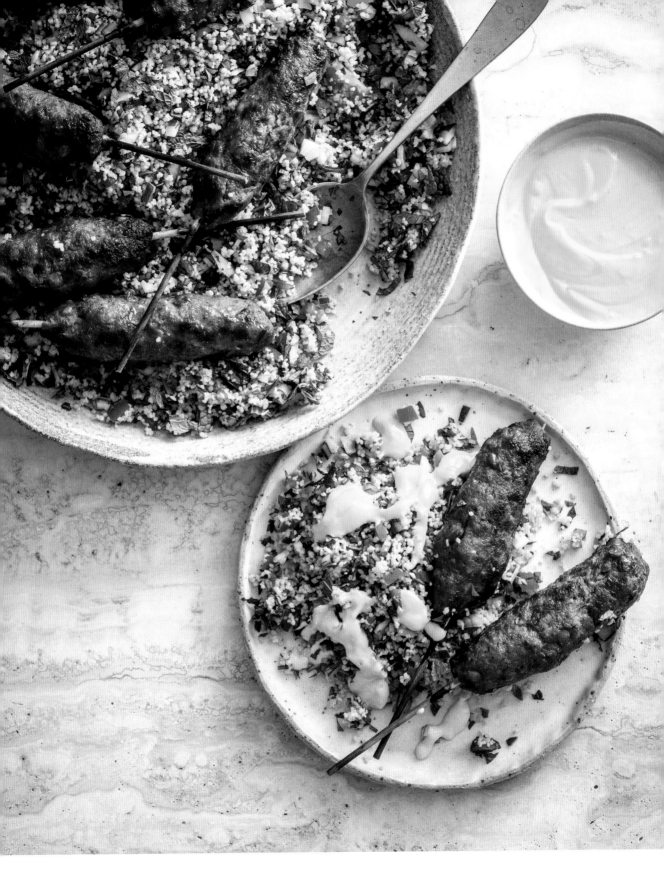

INFO PER SERVING: CALORIES 390 PROTEIN (G) 25 CARBS (G) 30 SUGAR (G) 11 FAT (G) 18 SATURATED FAT (G) 6.5 FIBRE (G) 6.5 SALT (G) 0.3

1 tbsp olive oil

1 onion, finely chopped

1 celery stick, finely chopped

1 carrot, finely chopped

250g chicken livers,
    finely sliced

2 garlic cloves, finely chopped

1 tsp dried sage

1 tbsp tomato purée

100ml marsala

250g cooked lentils (about
    100g uncooked weight)

300ml chicken stock

50g crème fraiche

400g pappardelle pasta

200g cavolo nero,
    de-stemmed and
    shredded (optional)

salt and black pepper

To serve
grated Parmesan (optional)

CHICKEN LIVER PASTA

Full of iron and vitamins, chicken livers are cheap and nutritious and make a fab sauce for pasta. Including some lentils helps balance out their richness. This dish is best made with flat noodles, such as tagliatelle or pappardelle, which hold the sauce well.

Heat the olive oil in a large, lidded sauté pan and add the onion, celery and carrot. Cook until softened and lightly coloured, then turn up the heat and add the chicken livers. Continue to cook, stirring regularly, until the livers are browned on all sides, then stir in the garlic and sage and cook for a further 2 minutes.

Add the tomato purée to the pan and cook for another couple of minutes, then add the marsala. Bring to the boil and stir to deglaze the pan. Stir in the cooked lentils, then pour in the chicken stock and season with salt and pepper.

Bring to the boil, then turn down to a simmer and leave until the sauce has reduced by about half – it should have a fairly thick texture. Stir in the crème fraiche.

While the sauce is cooking, bring a saucepan of water to the boil and add plenty of salt. Add the pasta and cook according to the packet instructions, adding the cavolo nero, if using, for the last 2 minutes.

Drain the pasta and serve with the sauce spooned over the top and some grated Parmesan, if using.

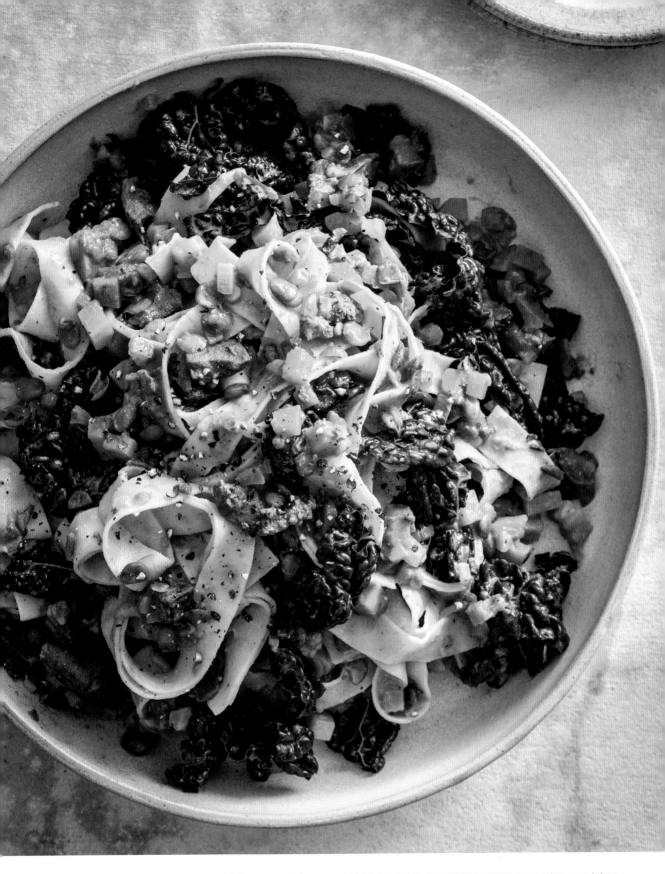

INFO PER SERVING: CALORIES 677 PROTEIN (G) 35 CARBS (G) 19 SUGAR (G) 10 FAT (G) 13 SATURATED FAT (G) 5 FIBRE (G) 13 SALT (G) 0.4

75g quinoa (or 225g cooked
  quinoa)

50g curly kale, stems removed

1 tsp olive oil

100g salad leaves (such as
  rocket, watercress and
  spinach)

200g mushrooms (such as
  chestnut), thickly sliced

200g cooked chicken,
  shredded

Dressing

2 tbsp olive oil

1 tsp sesame oil

1 tbsp soy sauce

juice of 1 lime

juice of 1 clementine
  or ½ orange

1 tbsp sushi ginger, finely
  chopped + 1 tbsp of
  the pickling liquor

¼ tsp ground allspice

¼ tsp Chinese five-spice
  powder

1 shallot, finely sliced

salt and black pepper

CHICKEN, MUSHROOM & QUINOA SALAD

Plenty of energy-giving protein in this dish as the quinoa, which is actually a seed not a grain, is a complete protein. If you have some chicken left over from a roast, this is the perfect way to use it and the special dressing really brings the salad to life.

First make the dressing. Whisk the oils with the soy sauce, lime and orange juice, sushi ginger and liquor and the spices. Season with salt and pepper and stir in the shallot.

Cook the quinoa according to the instructions on the packet. Next, massage the kale to soften it. Sprinkle the kale leaves with salt and the teaspoon of oil, then rub the leaves between your hands until the texture changes from firm and spiky to soft, slightly pliable and wet looking. Shred finely.

Arrange the salad leaves and quinoa over a platter. Toss the mushrooms in a couple of tablespoons of the dressing, then add these to the platter. Sprinkle over the kale, then top with the chicken. Drizzle over the remaining dressing and serve immediately.

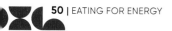

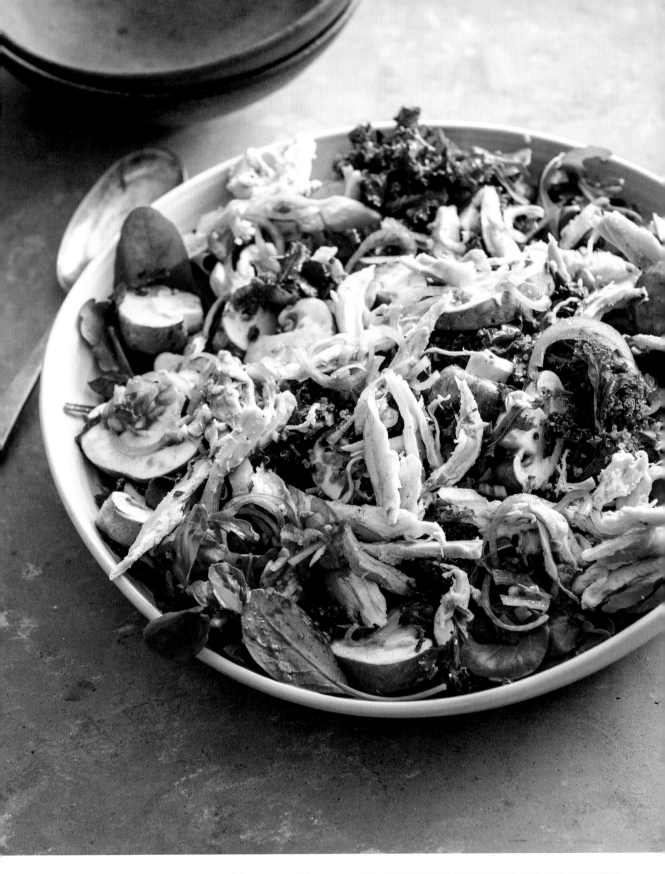

INFO PER SERVING: CALORIES 237 PROTEIN (G) 18.5 CARBS (G) 12 SUGAR (G) 3 FAT (G) 12 SATURATED FAT (G) 2 FIBRE (G) 3 SALT (G) 0.7

1 tbsp olive oil
1 small onion or 2 shallots,
    very finely chopped
500g mushrooms (we use
    a mixture of chestnut and
    shiitake), finely chopped
leaves from 3 tarragon sprigs,
    finely chopped
leaves from a small thyme
    sprig, finely chopped
2 garlic cloves, finely chopped
2 tsp mustard (tarragon if you
    have it, otherwise Dijon)
100g ricotta or cream cheese
squeeze of lemon or lime juice
salt and black pepper

To serve
wholegrain crackers

MUSHROOM & TARRAGON PÂTÉ

This is a really handy little treat to have in the fridge for when you feel like a snack and it's lovely served with crackers and some raw veg. If you want a change from the mustard, you could add some chilli flakes or paprika instead.

Heat the olive oil in a large frying pan. Add the onion or shallots and cook over a medium to high heat until lightly browned, then add the mushrooms. Season with salt and pepper, then cook, stirring regularly, until the mushrooms have reduced down and the pan is quite dry. The mushrooms will give out a lot of liquid initially, but this should evaporate away.

Stir in the herbs and garlic and cook for another couple of minutes. Remove the pan from the heat and stir in the mustard.

Transfer everything to a food processor or blender and process until the mixture is well broken down. Add the ricotta or cream cheese and continue to process until just slightly textured or smooth, as you prefer. Taste for seasoning and add a squeeze of lemon or lime juice. Transfer to a container and chill for an hour. Serve with crackers.

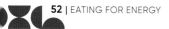

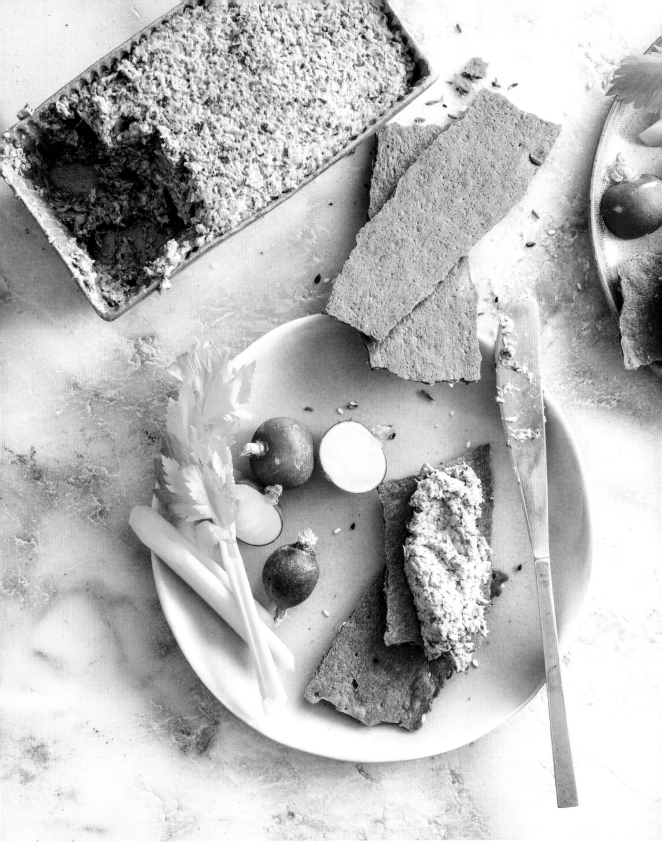

INFO PER SERVING (WITH WHOLEGRAIN CRACKERS):   CALORIES 105   PROTEIN (G) 5   CARBS (G) 9   SUGAR (G) 2   FAT (G) 5.5   SATURATED FAT (G) 2

FIBRE (G) 1.5   SALT (G) 0.3

1 tin of anchovies

1 leek, finely sliced

3 courgettes, sliced

3 garlic cloves, crushed

½ tsp dried oregano

2 x 400g cans of white beans

juice and zest of 1 lemon

a few basil leaves, torn

salt and black pepper

BRAISED WHITE BEANS WITH ANCHOVIES, LEEKS & COURGETTES

You might be surprised at the anchovies in this recipe, but they just add a savoury richness to the dish, rather than a strong anchovy flavour. Borlotti or butter beans instead of cannellini are also good and you might like to serve a tomato and red onion salad on the side as a nice contrast. Simple and really tasty.

Tip the anchovies and their oil into a saucepan. Place over a gentle heat, then break up the anchovies with a wooden spoon until they dissolve into the oil – this should happen quite quickly.

Add the leek and courgettes. Stir to combine and then add a splash of water. Cover the pan and leave the vegetables to braise for about 10 minutes, stirring regularly, until they are on the tender side of al dente.

Add the garlic and oregano and continue to cook for another minute or so, then stir in the beans, lemon juice and zest. Taste for seasoning and add black pepper and salt if necessary. Heat for another few minutes until the beans are warmed through, then garnish with basil leaves.

Serve in shallow bowls or piled onto sourdough toast.

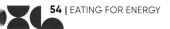

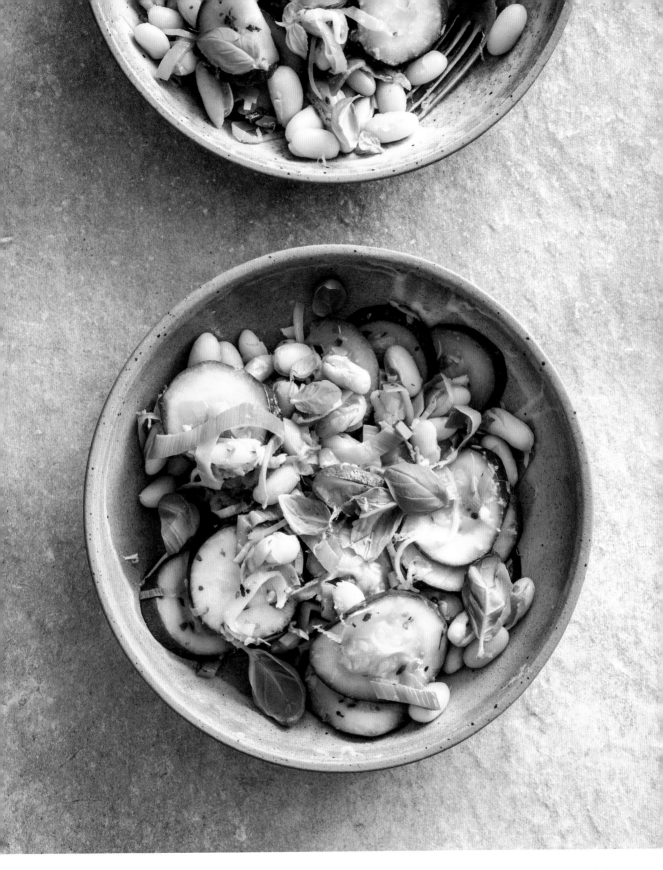

INFO PER SERVING: CALORIES 163 PROTEIN (G) 12 CARBS (G) 19 SUGAR (G) 4 FAT (G) 2 SATURATED FAT (G) 0.5 FIBRE (G) 10.5 SALT (G) 1.2

Serves: **4**   Prep: **10 minutes**   Cooking time: **1 hour 10 minutes**

4 sweet potatoes

1 tbsp olive oil

200g feta

25g sun-blushed or
   sun-dried tomatoes

½ tsp dried oregano

½ tsp hot paprika

salt and black pepper

Spinach

1 tbsp olive oil

1 small red onion, finely
   chopped

1 hot red chilli, finely chopped

1 garlic clove, finely chopped

150g baby spinach

squeeze of lemon or lime juice

BAKED SWEET POTATOES WITH FETA & SPINACH

Keep the cooking of the spinach to a minimum here to help preserve the B vitamins – cook just until it's wilted down but still fresh and green. We've learned to add a little lemon juice to our spinach, as vitamin C helps the body absorb iron from vegetables.

Preheat the oven to 200°C/Fan 180°C/Gas 6. Pierce the sweet potatoes all over with a skewer and make a deep incision down the centre of each one. Rub them with olive oil and sprinkle with salt. Place the potatoes in a roasting tin and bake in the oven for 40–45 minutes or until cooked through.

Crumble up the feta and put it in a food processor with the tomatoes, oregano and paprika. Season with plenty of black pepper and process until smooth. Break or cut the sweet potatoes open without splitting them completely in half and divide the feta mixture between them. Put the potatoes back in the oven for a 10–15 minutes until the feta is soft and lightly browned on top.

To prepare the spinach, heat the olive oil in a large frying pan and add the onion and chilli. Sauté until the onion is translucent, then add the garlic and stir for another couple of minutes. Add the spinach and stir-fry until it has wilted down but is still fresh and green and hasn't completely lost its shape. Be careful, as it will be quite bulky and you don't want it to spill out of the pan. Season with salt and pepper and squeeze over the lemon or lime juice.

Pile the spinach mixture on top of the sweet potatoes and serve immediately.

 Tip: If you're making this recipe, put an extra potato in the oven so you can bake the sweet potato bread on page 30.

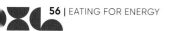

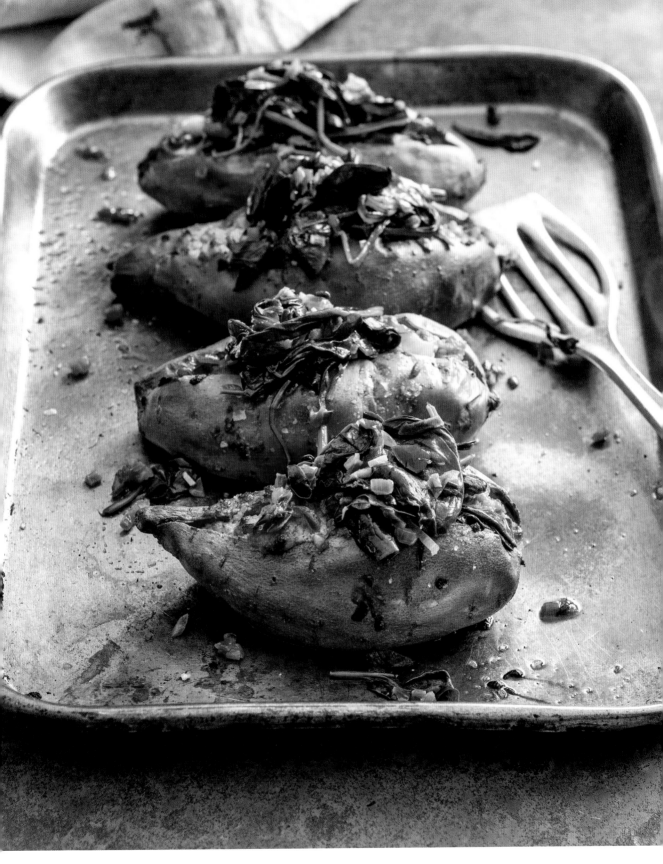

INFO PER SERVING: CALORIES 485 PROTEIN (G) 12.5 CARBS (G) 64.5 SUGAR (G) 19 FAT (G) 17 SATURATED FAT (G) 8 FIBRE (G) 11 SALT (G) 1.7

2 tbsp olive oil

400g lamb mince

1 large onion, finely chopped

2 celery sticks, finely chopped

2 large carrots, coarsely grated

1 large beetroot, coarsely grated

3 garlic cloves, finely chopped

needles from a rosemary sprig, finely chopped

1 tsp dried oregano

100ml red wine (optional)

400g can of chopped tomatoes

250ml lamb, chicken or vegetable stock

salt and black pepper

Topping

1 tbsp olive oil

1 large cauliflower (800g–1kg), finely chopped

1 tbsp crème fraiche or soured cream

a few dill sprigs, finely chopped

50g Cheddar or other hard cheese, grated (optional)

SHEPHERD'S PIE WITH CAULIFLOWER MASH

We always love a shepherd's pie and this version has a beautiful cauliflower topping as a change from regular mash. The method we've suggested for cooking the cauliflower gives a nice creamy, result and means it's less likely to be waterlogged than if it's boiled or steamed in the usual way.

First start the filling. Heat a tablespoon of the olive oil in a large frying pan. Add the lamb mince and fry it over a high heat until browned. Remove with a slotted spoon and drain on kitchen paper.

Heat the remaining tablespoon of oil in a large saucepan and add the onion, celery, carrots and beetroot. Sauté for 5 minutes until the veg are just starting to soften, then add the garlic, rosemary and oregano and stir for another minute. Add the browned lamb mince, pour in the red wine, if using, and bring to the boil. Simmer until most of the wine has boiled off before adding the tomatoes and stock. (If not using the red wine, just add the tomatoes and stock after the mince.) Season with salt and pepper, bring to the boil, then turn down and simmer for 20 minutes.

To make the topping, heat the oil in a large lidded pan. Add the cauliflower and sauté over a high heat until it starts to look slightly transparent. Add a splash of water and season with salt. Put a lid on the pan and leave the cauli to gently steam for about 5 minutes until tender. Remove from the heat and drain the cauliflower, then mash it thoroughly. This is best done with a stick blender, but a traditional masher works too. Stir through the crème fraiche or soured cream and the dill.

Preheat the oven to 200°C/Fan 180°C/Gas 6. Pile the filling into a large ovenproof dish, then spoon over the cauliflower topping. Make sure the filling is completely covered, especially around the edges. Sprinkle with the grated cheese, if using, and place in the oven.

Cook in the oven for 25–30 minutes until the filling is bubbling under the cauliflower and the top has lightly browned. Serve with a salad or some green veg.

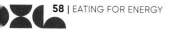

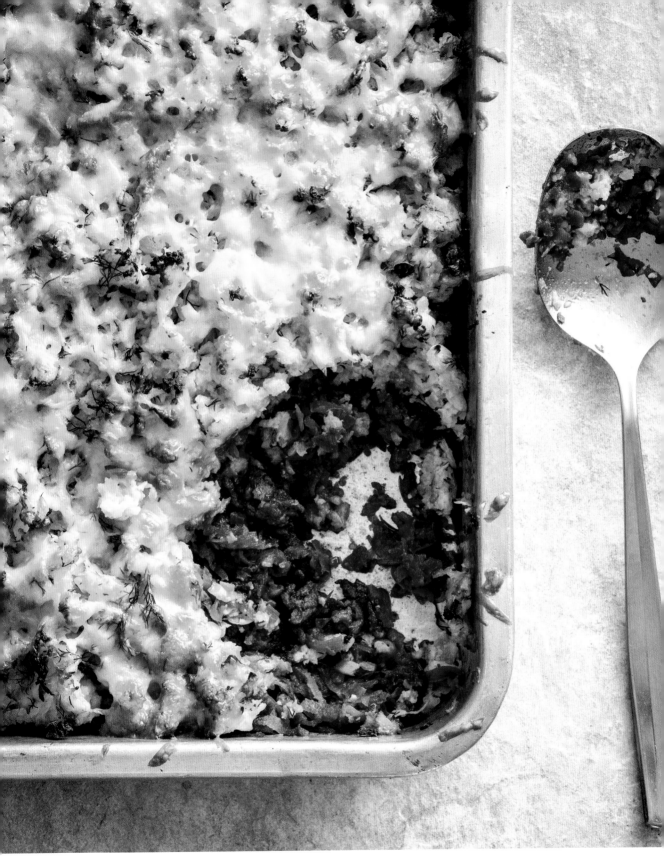

INFO PER SERVING: CALORIES 438 PROTEIN (G) 28 CARBS (G) 19 SUGAR (G) 15 FAT (G) 24 SATURATED FAT (G) 8.5 FIBRE (G) 7 SALT (G) 0.4

100g nut butter

50g honey

75g dates, very finely chopped

2 balls of stem ginger, very
    finely chopped

a few drops of vanilla extract

100g oats

25g cocoa powder

25g sesame seeds

½ tsp ground cinnamon

large pinch of chilli powder

pinch of salt

To coat

cocoa powder

DATE & GINGER ENERGY BALLS

No, these are not a comedy act in a northern nightclub but real little power houses which provide a healthy pick-me-up when you feel in need of an energy boost. If you fancy, replace some of the oats with desiccated coconut. Pop a couple of these in your lunchbox and you'll thank us.

Put the nut butter, honey, dates, stem ginger and vanilla in a small saucepan. Heat gently to melt everything together, pressing down on the dates with the back of a spoon to make sure they break up well with everything else. Remove from the heat.

Put the oats in a food processor and pulse a few times to break them up a bit. Don't go crazy when you do this, as you don't want the oats to be as fine as oatmeal. Put the oats in a bowl with all the remaining ingredients and mix. Add the mixture to the saucepan and stir thoroughly to combine, then – messy, but necessary – knead with your hands to help everything come together.

Divide the mixture into 16 and roll into balls. Dust lightly with cocoa powder and store in an airtight container in the fridge.

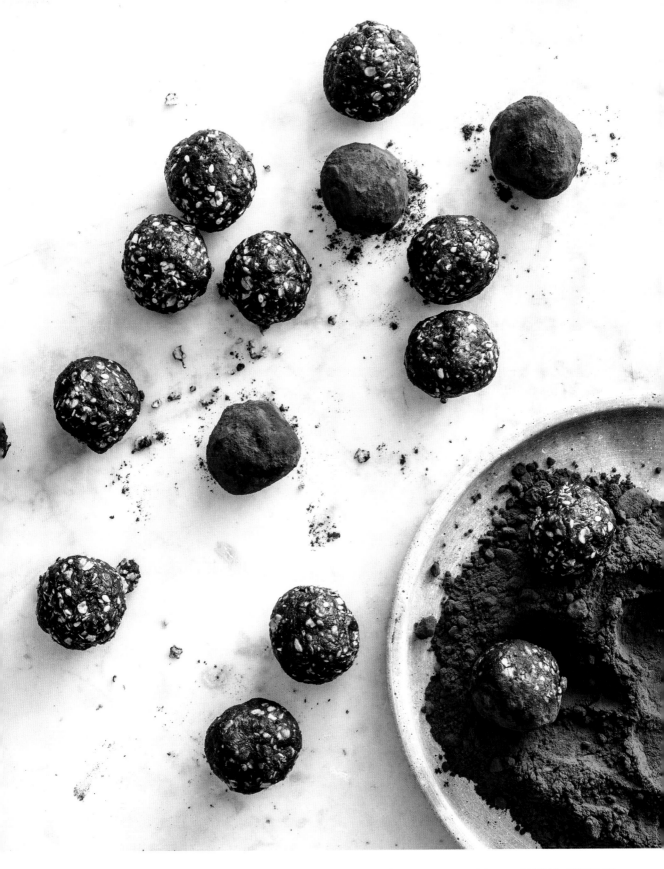

INFO PER BALL: CALORIES 95   PROTEIN (G) 3   CARBS (G) 9   SUGAR (G) 4.5   FAT (G) 5   SATURATED FAT (G) 1.5   FIBRE (G) 1.5   SALT (G) 1.5

FIVE A DAY

We all know we should be eating at least five portions of fruit and veg a day and now we hear that the nutrition experts are advising us to aim for even more – ten a day if you can. Don't forget that canned, dried and frozen vegetables all count – and can sometimes be cheaper than fresh – so make sure you have staples like peas, spinach and sweetcorn in your freezer to add to dishes, and cans of beans and tomatoes in your cupboard. They're great for quick meals or for bulking out a soup or tray bake. Variety is key too, so don't just stick to the same veg every week – branch out and try some less familiar ones. In Japan, they advise having five colours of veg on your plate to get the range of nutrients you need, so think rainbow when planning your meal.

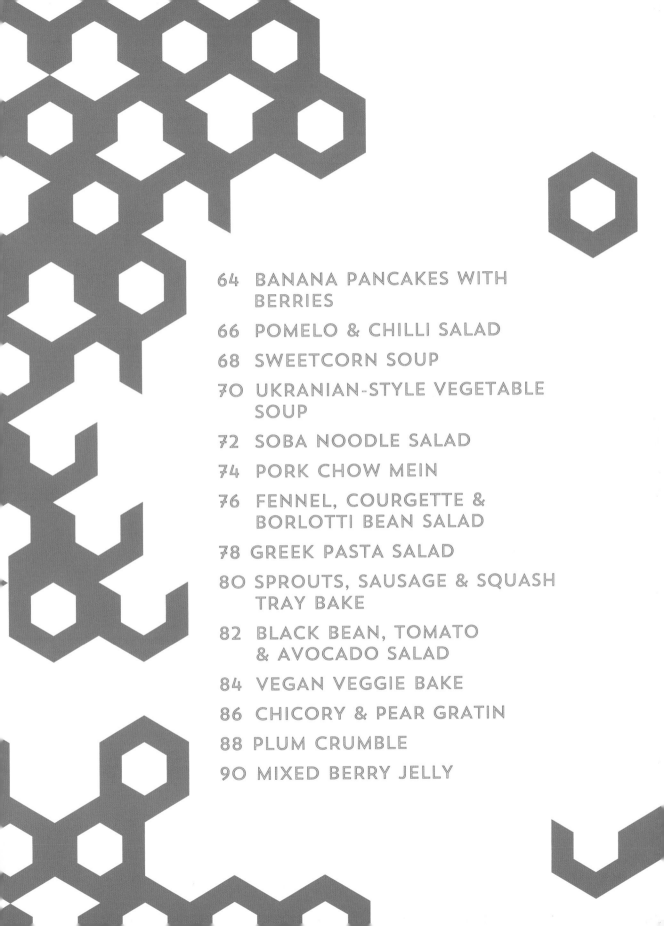

100g raisins or sultanas

150g wholemeal flour
(spelt works well)

2 tsp baking powder

½ tsp bicarbonate of soda

½ tsp ground cinnamon

pinch of salt

2 bananas, mashed

1 egg

125ml milk

1 tbsp yoghurt or kefir

zest of 1 lime

oil or butter, for frying

To serve

maple syrup or honey

400g berries

yoghurt or crème fraiche

BANANA PANCAKES WITH BERRIES

Light and fluffy, these pancakes are still beautifully sustaining. Served with some fresh berries and yoghurt or crème fraiche, they make a great start to your day.

Put the raisins or sultanas in a small saucepan and just cover with water (about 100ml). Bring to the boil and leave to simmer until most of the water has been absorbed. Remove the pan from the heat and leave to cool.

Put the flour in a large bowl with the baking powder, bicarbonate of soda, cinnamon and a generous pinch of salt.

Put the bananas in another bowl and beat in the egg, milk, yoghurt or kefir and the lime zest. Add this mixture to the dry ingredients and whisk to form a thick batter. Stir in the dried fruit.

Heat a large frying pan and rub the base with a little oil or butter. Add heaped tablespoons of the batter to the pan – you should be able to make 4 pancakes at a time. When the undersides are cooked and bubbles start to appear on the surface, flip the pancakes over. They will be quite fragile, so do this carefully. When they're cooked through, remove and keep warm. Cook the remaining batter the same way.

Serve with a drizzle of maple syrup or honey, the berries and spoonfuls of yoghurt or crème fraiche.

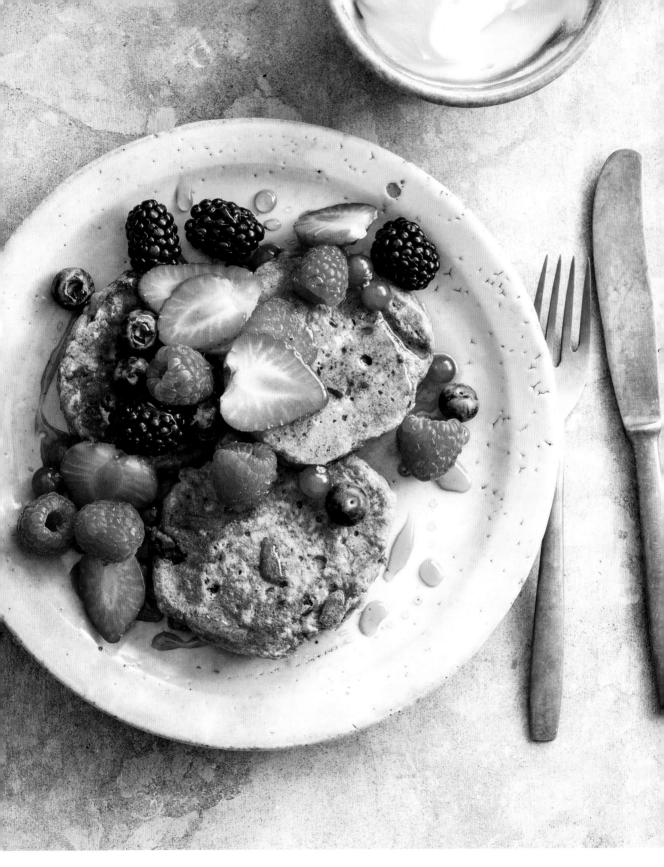

INFO PER SERVING: CALORIES 341 PROTEIN (G) 10 CARBS (G) 61 SUGAR (G) 34 FAT (G) 4.5 SATURATED FAT (G) 2 FIBRE (G) 8 SALT (G) 1.7

1 red onion, finely sliced

1 tbsp rice vinegar

½ small cauliflower, cut into
small florets

2 tbsp desiccated coconut

1 pomelo (see method) or
1 large grapefruit

2 red chillies, finely chopped

½ cucumber, diced

150g baby corn, cut into
rounds

100g radishes, cut into rounds

50g rocket, roughly chopped

1 small bunch of coriander,
chopped

leaves from a small bunch
of mint, finely chopped

1 tbsp sesame seeds

salt and black pepper

Dressing

1 tbsp fish sauce

zest and juice of 1 lime

1 tsp runny honey

POMELO & CHILLI SALAD

Pomelos are quite widely available now, but you could also use grapefruit for this salad if you prefer. Fresh and crunchy with all the veg chopped quite small, this makes a great lunch – and it's good for vegans if you use soy sauce instead of fish sauce.

Put the red onion slices in a small bowl and sprinkle with salt. Add the rice vinegar and leave to stand while you prepare everything else.

Bring a pan of water to the boil, then add the cauliflower florets. Bring back to the boil, then drain and refresh the florets under cold water.

Spread the coconut evenly over a dry frying pan. Toast the coconut over a medium heat until very lightly browned, then tip it into a bowl to cool.

To prepare the pomelo or grapefruit, cut the peel and pith away in wedges, then remove any pith and membrane from the flesh. Pull the flesh into bite-sized clumps.

To assemble the salad, strain the onion, reserving the vinegar. Whisk the vinegar with the remaining dressing ingredients and taste. Add salt and pepper and more honey as needed.

Gently toss all the vegetables and herbs together in the dressing, then divide between 4 bowls. Sprinkle with the coconut and sesame seeds before serving.

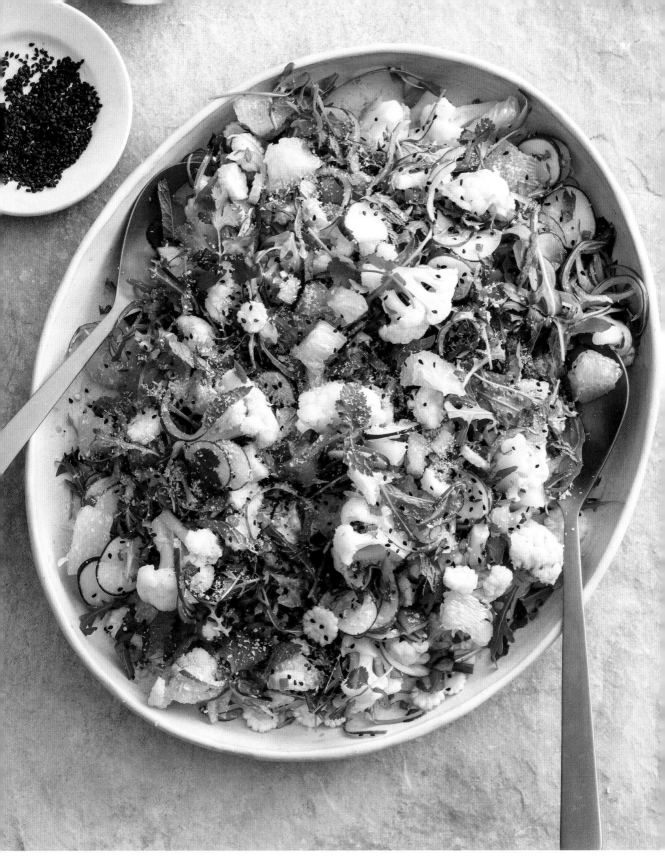

INFO PER SERVING: CALORIES 167 PROTEIN (G) 7 CARBS (G) 14 SUGAR (G) 12 FAT (G) 8 SATURATED FAT (G) 4.5 FIBRE (G) 6 SALT (G) 2.1

1 tbsp olive oil

1 onion, chopped

2 celery sticks, finely chopped

½ large red pepper or 1 small, diced

1 medium floury potato, diced (no need to peel)

100g squash, peeled and diced

250g cauliflower, chopped

2 garlic cloves, finely chopped

1 tsp sweet paprika

½ tsp fennel seeds

800ml vegetable stock

400g sweetcorn (defrosted if frozen)

100g fresh tomatoes (preferably orange or yellow)

salt and black pepper

Garnish (optional)

1 tsp olive oil

25g pumpkin seeds

½ tsp paprika

SWEETCORN SOUP

There's a whole galaxy of veg in this pot of soup which is great, as the experts tell us we should be eating a good range of colourful vegetables for their different nutrients. And we urge you to try the pumpkin seed garnish. These little beauties might be tiny but they pack a massive nutritional punch.

Heat the olive oil in a large saucepan. Add the onion, celery, red pepper, potato, squash and cauliflower and sauté them over a medium-high heat until the onion is starting to look translucent.

Stir in the garlic, sweet paprika and fennel seeds and season with plenty of salt and pepper. Stir for another minute or so, then pour in the vegetable stock and add half the sweetcorn. Bring to the boil and simmer for 5 minutes.

Purée the remaining sweetcorn and the fresh tomatoes in a food processor or a blender, adding a splash of the liquid from the soup to help it along. When the mixture is smooth, add it to the soup and continue to cook until the vegetables are very soft. This will take at least another 15 minutes. Keep an eye on the thickness and add a little more stock if necessary. Check the seasoning and add salt and black pepper to taste.

For the garnish, if using, heat the olive oil in a small frying pan. Add the pumpkin seeds, paprika and plenty of salt and pepper. Stir until the pumpkin seeds are lightly toasted, then tip them on to a plate to cool. Ladle the soup into bowls and top with the pumpkin seeds.

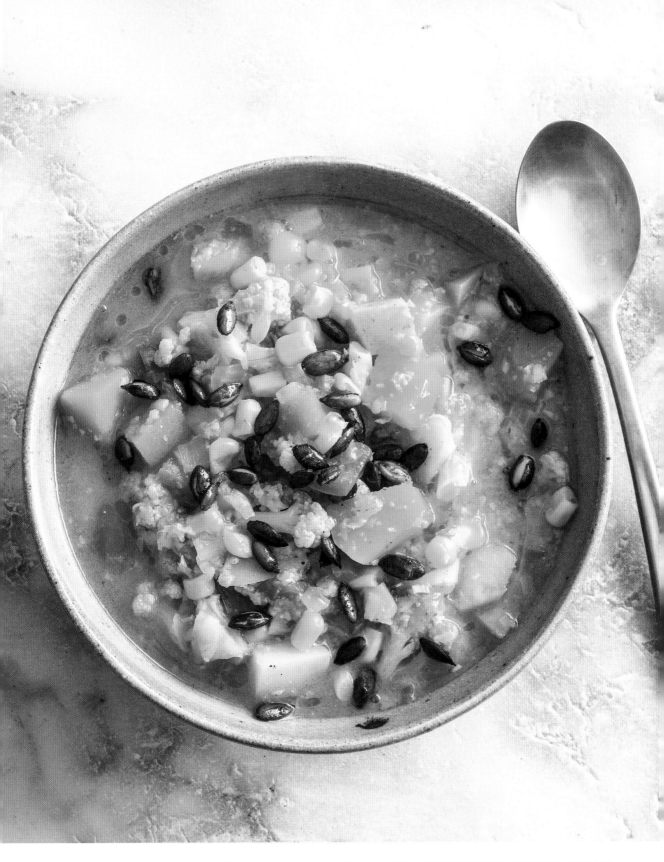

INFO PER SERVING: CALORIES 194 PROTEIN (G) 7 CARBS (G) 25 SUGAR (G) 10 FAT (G) 6 SATURATED FAT (G) 1 FIBRE (G) 7 SALT (G) 0.2

2 tbsp olive oil

1 large onion, finely chopped

2 celery sticks, diced

400g root vegetables (carrot,
turnip, celeriac, beetroot),
diced

½ red cabbage, chopped

100g smoked ham or sausage,
finely chopped (optional)

3 tbsp tomato purée

1 tsp ground allspice

2 bay leaves

1.2 litres vegetable or chicken
stock

2 large gherkins, finely diced,
plus some of the pickle brine
(pickle brine optional)

3 tbsp pitted olives (black
or green), sliced

salt and black pepper

Garnish

small bunch of dill,
finely chopped

a few parsley sprigs,
finely chopped

soured cream, live yoghurt
or kefir

UKRANIAN-STYLE VEGETABLE SOUP

We've based this recipe on a classic Ukranian dish – solyanka. It's a bit like minestrone in that you can add all sorts of veggies or meat to it, but the special feature is the addition of olives and gherkins which bring a nice zesty blast of flavour. We've suggested smoked ham or sausage but you could use any cured meat.

Heat the olive oil in a large saucepan. Add the onion, celery and root vegetables and sauté over a high heat for 5 minutes until the veg are starting to take on some colour round the edges. Add the cabbage and the ham or sausage, if using, and sauté for another few minutes.

Add the tomato purée and allspice and stir until all the vegetables are coated and you can smell that the tomato purée is cooked. Add the bay leaves and pour in the stock, then season with salt and pepper.

Bring to the boil, then turn down the heat and leave to simmer for about 20 minutes until the vegetables are tender.

Stir in the gherkins and olives and simmer for another minute or so. Taste – if you want the flavour to be slightly more sour, add some of the pickle brine. Serve garnished with the herbs and either the soured cream, yoghurt or kefir.

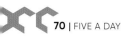

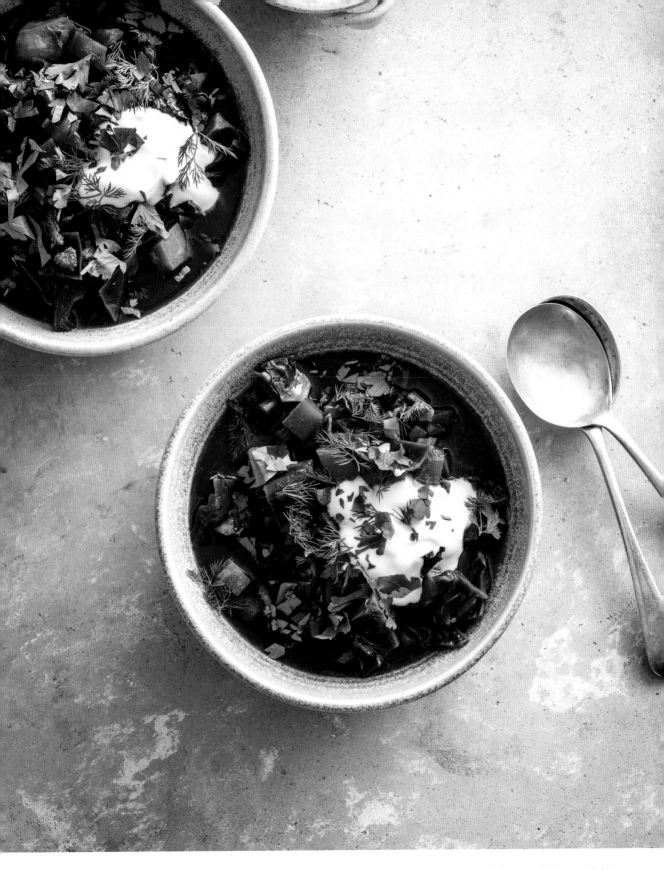

INFO PER SERVING: CALORIES 231 PROTEIN (G) 10 CARBS (G) 18 SUGAR (G) 14.5 FAT (G) 11 SATURATED FAT (G) 2 FIBRE (G) 10 SALT (G) 1.4

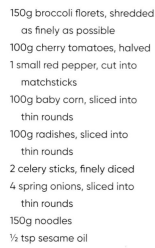

150g broccoli florets, shredded
as finely as possible

100g cherry tomatoes, halved

1 small red pepper, cut into
matchsticks

100g baby corn, sliced into
thin rounds

100g radishes, sliced into
thin rounds

2 celery sticks, finely diced

4 spring onions, sliced into
thin rounds

150g noodles

½ tsp sesame oil

salt and black pepper

Dressing

zest and juice of 1 lime

1 hot chilli, finely chopped

2 tbsp fish sauce

½ tsp sugar

¼ tsp turmeric

Garnish

small bunch of coriander,
finely chopped

1 tsp sesame seeds

2 tbsp peanuts, toasted and
lightly crushed

SOBA NOODLE SALAD

Cooked and cooled noodles here provide resistant starch which is a fibre that's super-good for your gut. And there are loads of vegetables to make this a healthy, satisfying feast to delight you. This is dead easy to prepare, but you do need to allow time to salt the broccoli and for the dressed salad to absorb the flavours. It's a great one to prepare for your lunch box the next day.

Sprinkle the broccoli florets with half a teaspoon of salt and leave them in a colander for half an hour. Give them a quick rinse under the cold tap, then put them in a bowl with the rest of the vegetables.

Cook the noodles according to the packet instructions, then toss them in the sesame oil and add them to the bowl.

Whisk all the dressing ingredients together with a generous grinding of black pepper and some salt. Pour the dressing over the salad and toss thoroughly. Leave to stand for half an hour.

Serve garnished with the coriander, sesame seeds and peanuts.

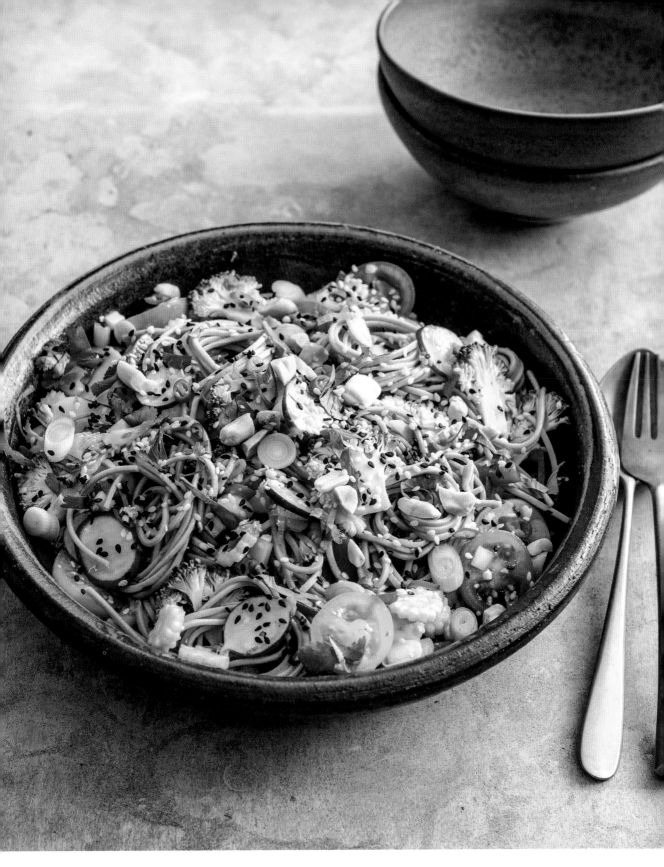

INFO PER SERVING: CALORIES 173 PROTEIN (G) 7 CARBS (G) 30 SUGAR (G) 5 FAT (G) 1.5 SATURATED FAT (G) 0.5 FIBRE (G) 4.5 SALT (G) 0.9

150g green beans, trimmed
and halved

120g dried noodles

2 tbsp vegetable or olive oil

300g pork mince

1 large carrot, cut into
matchsticks

1 red pepper, finely sliced

½ small white or green pointed
cabbage, finely shredded

150g baby corn, quartered
lengthways into strips

50g frozen peas, defrosted

Sauce

1 tsp sesame oil

2 tbsp soy sauce

1 tbsp mirin

1 tbsp rice vinegar

2 tbsp kecap manis

2 garlic cloves, crushed

10g root ginger, grated

100ml chicken or vegetable
stock

2 tsp cornflour (optional)

salt and black pepper

Garnish

4 spring onions, halved and
shredded

small bunch of coriander,
finely chopped

1 tsp sesame seeds

PORK CHOW MEIN

Yum – this is really moreish, the kind of dish you just can't stop eating. It's packed with veg and so is really healthy but also totally delicious with bags of flavour and texture. No need for a takeaway when you can make this! We like to use flat wholemeal noodles rather than nested, but that's up to you.

For the sauce, simply put everything in a bowl and whisk together. Taste and add salt and pepper as necessary. If you want a thicker sauce, add 2 teaspoons of cornflour.

Bring a pan of water to the boil, add the green beans and cook for 1 minute. Drain and refresh under cold water. Cook the noodles according to the packet instructions and set aside.

Heat half the oil in a wok – when the air above the oil starts to shimmer, it's hot enough. Add the pork and stir-fry until well browned. Pour the sauce into the wok and keep it over a high heat until the pork has cooked through and the liquid has reduced and thickened. Tip everything into a bowl, then wipe over the wok with kitchen paper.

Heat the remaining oil in the wok. Add all the vegetables, including the green beans, and stir-fry for several minutes until they have collapsed down a bit and are just al dente. Put the pork and sauce back in the wok, along with the noodles, and carefully stir everything together, making sure it's all piping hot. Taste and add more soy sauce if you think it necessary.

Divide the contents of the wok between 4 bowls and garnish with the spring onions, coriander and sesame seeds.

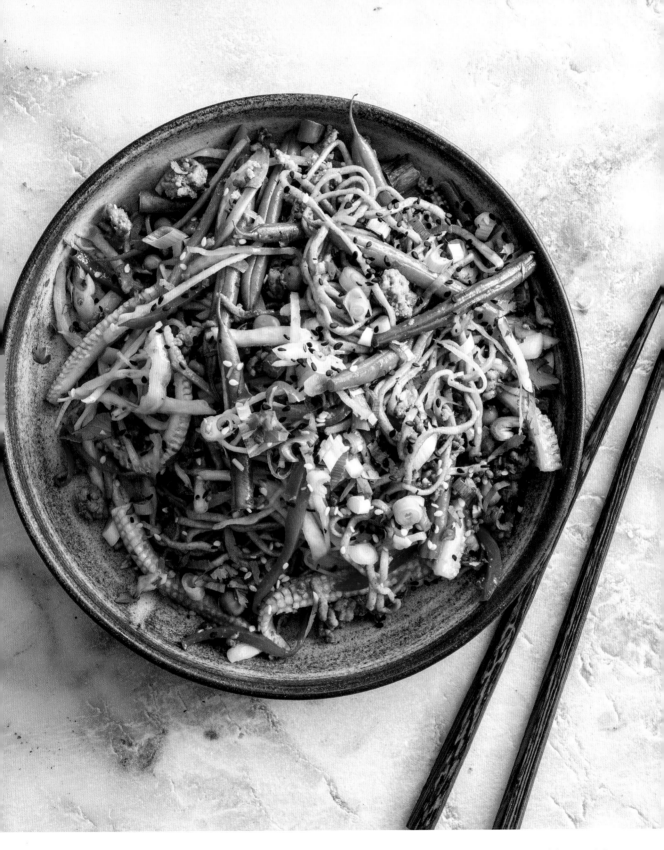

INFO PER SERVING: CALORIES 400 PROTEIN (G) 24 CARBS (G) 37 SUGAR (G) 12 FAT (G) 16 SATURATED FAT (G) 3.5 FIBRE (G) 8 SALT (G) 3

FENNEL, COURGETTE & BORLOTTI BEAN SALAD

1 small red onion, sliced

1 large courgette, thinly sliced on the diagonal

1 tbsp olive oil

½ tsp mixed herbs

100g rocket leaves

400g can of borlotti beans, drained and rinsed

1 large fennel bulb, trimmed and very finely sliced

1 orange, segmented (peel and central membrane reserved)

salt and black pepper

Dressing

2 tbsp olive oil

leaves from a small bunch of basil

juice from the orange skin and central membrane (see above)

juice of 1 lemon

1 tsp balsamic vinegar

pinch of chilli powder or flakes

Garnish

leaves from a thyme sprig

a few mint leaves

1 tbsp flaked almonds, toasted

The secret of a great salad is to make a tantalising combo of flavours and textures and that's what this is. We didn't set out to make this vegan but it really works, and if you're not vegan you could garnish it with Parmesan shavings instead of almonds.

Put the onion slices in a bowl of cold salted water and leave to soak for half an hour while you prepare the rest of the vegetables.

Heat a griddle pan until it's too hot to hold your hand over. Toss the courgette slices in the oil and mixed herbs and season with salt and pepper. Grill the slices on both sides until softened and char lines have developed, then remove and set them aside to cool.

Arrange the rocket over a serving dish and sprinkle over the beans, fennel and grilled courgettes. Drain the onion slices and sprinkle them over too, then top with the orange segments.

For the dressing, put the olive oil and basil leaves in a small food processor and squeeze in any juice from the orange peel and membrane. Add the lemon juice, vinegar and chilli, then season with salt and pepper. Blend to a fairly smooth, green-flecked dressing.

Drizzle the dressing over the salad and toss very gently to combine. Garnish with the thyme, mint and flaked almonds, then serve immediately.

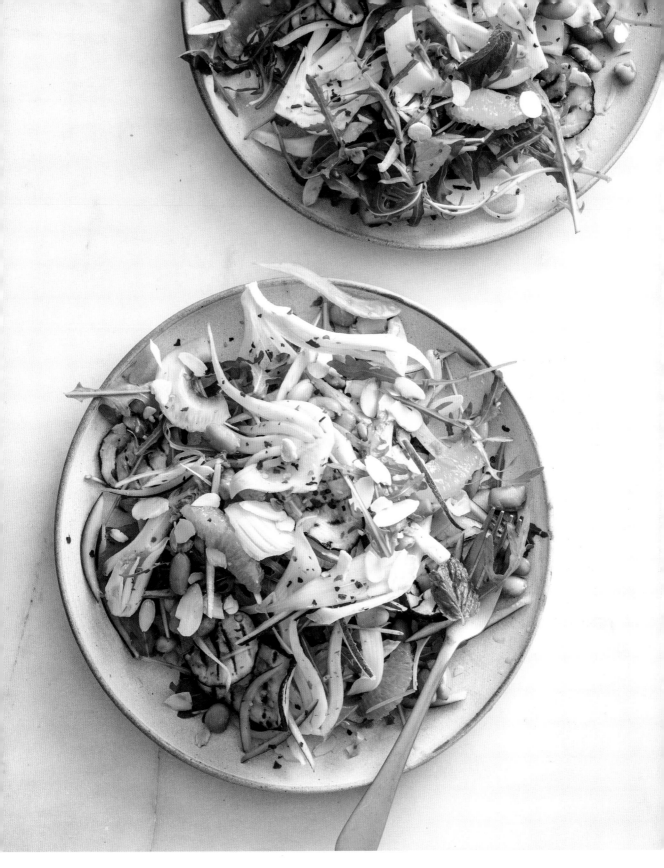

INFO PER SERVING: CALORIES 230 PROTEIN (G) 10 CARBS (G) 13 SUGAR (G) 8 FAT (G) 12 SATURATED FAT (G) 1.5 FIBRE (G) 16 SALT (G) 0.1

150g short pasta

1 red onion, sliced into
    crescents

250g cherry tomatoes, halved

2 tbsp olive oil

1 tbsp red wine vinegar

1 tsp dried oregano

50g rocket, roughly chopped

½ cucumber, diced

1 green pepper, finely diced

100g pitted black olives,
    halved

200g feta, cubed

salt and black pepper

To serve

zest of 1 lemon

olive oil

red wine vinegar

leaves from a small bunch
    of fresh oregano

GREEK PASTA SALAD

We love a Greek salad and this combines those lovely flavours with some pasta to make a heartier dish to enjoy for lunch or supper. Grilling the tomatoes makes them into more of a sauce than a dressing and the cooked and cooled pasta gives you gut-friendly resistant starch. This is a great lunch box dish.

Cook the pasta in plenty of salted boiling water until al dente, then drain and set aside to cool. Soak the onion slices in a bowl of cold salted water.

Heat the grill to its highest setting. Put the cherry tomatoes in an ovenproof dish and drizzle over the olive oil and red wine vinegar. Sprinkle over the oregano. Put the dish under the grill until the tomatoes have softened and have taken on some colour, then leave to cool to room temperature.

Put the cooled pasta in a bowl with the tomatoes and any juices from the oven dish and mix thoroughly. Add the rocket, cucumber, green pepper, black olives, drained red onion slices and feta, then season with salt and pepper.

Stir very gently to combine – you don't want the feta to break up too much – then grate over the lemon zest. Taste and add a little more olive oil and red wine vinegar if you think the salad needs it. Garnish with the fresh oregano.

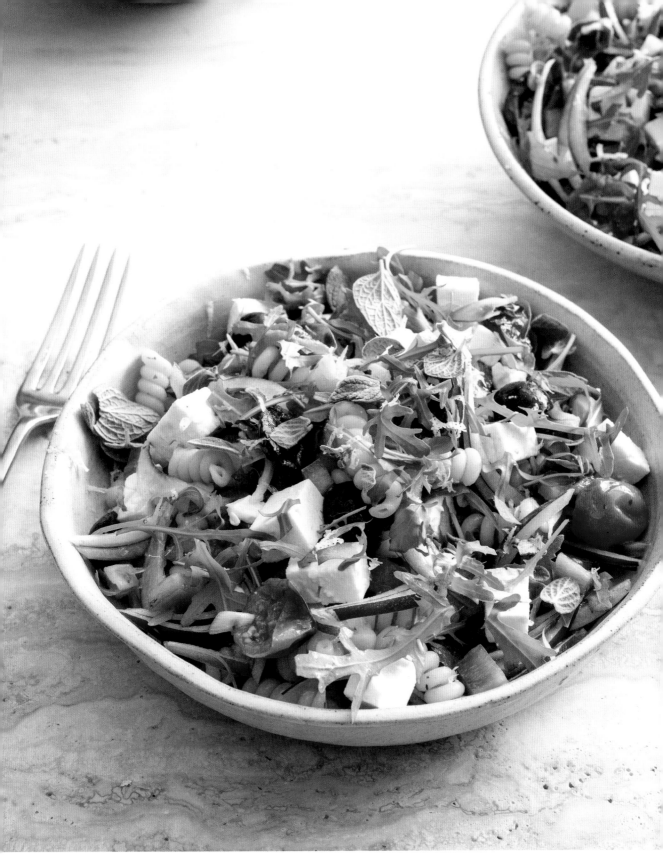

INFO PER SERVING: CALORIES 440   PROTEIN (G) 15   CARBS (G) 39   SUGAR (G) 7.   FAT (G) 24   SATURATED FAT (G) 9   FIBRE (G) 5.5   SALT (G) 2

3 red onions, cut into wedges

½ medium squash, cut into 8 wedges (no need to peel)

2 tbsp olive oil

6 sausages, skinned

500g Brussels sprouts, trimmed but left whole

100ml red wine or chicken stock

3 tsp maple syrup

1 tbsp tomato purée

1 tsp dried sage

2 garlic cloves, finely chopped

salt and black pepper

SPROUTS, SAUSAGE & SQUASH TRAY BAKE

We always love a tray bake, especially when there are sausages in it. Here, the sausages add extra flavour to a great selection of vegetables and the sprouts give the dish a hint of a festive feel – after all, a sprout is for life, not just for Christmas! The skin of some varieties of squash can be eaten and provides extra fibre and we suggest roasting with the skin on anyway, as it's so much easier to remove once cooked.

Preheat the oven to 200°C/Fan 180°C/Gas 6.

Put the red onion wedges and squash in a bowl and season with salt and pepper. Drizzle with a tablespoon of the olive oil and toss to combine, then arrange them evenly over a large roasting tray.

Divide each sausage into 3 pieces and roll them into balls. Dot these over the onion and squash. Put the tray in the oven and roast for 20 minutes.

Meanwhile, steam the sprouts over simmering water for up to 10 minutes, checking them after 6 minutes. They should be al dente, not soft. Remove the sprouts from the steamer and, using the back of a frying pan or saucepan, squash each one gently so it breaks open.

Whisk the red wine or chicken stock with 50ml of water, 2 teaspoons of the maple syrup, the tomato purée, sage and garlic. Pour this mixture around the contents of the roasting tin. Toss the sprouts with the remaining olive oil, then brush with the rest of the maple syrup. Add them to the roasting tin and roast for a further 20 minutes. Remove from the oven and serve immediately.

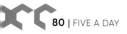

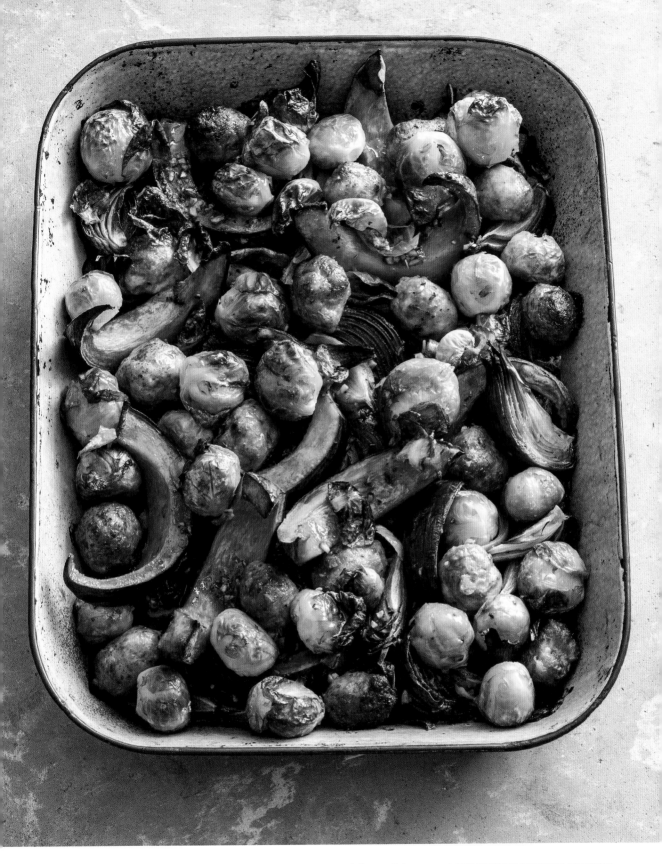

INFO PER SERVING: CALORIES 457 PROTEIN (G) 28.5 CARBS (G) 20.5 SUGAR (G) 16 FAT (G) 24.5 SATURATED FAT (G) 7.5 FIBRE (G) 11 SALT (G) 1.3

1 red onion, finely sliced

1 avocado, flesh diced

zest and juice of 1 lime

100g watercress or similar
    salad leaves

400g can of black beans,
    drained

2 celery sticks, very finely sliced

250g tomatoes (mixed if
    possible), roughly chopped

coriander, mint and basil
    leaves

2 tbsp pumpkin seeds

salt and black pepper

Dressing

50g tomatoes

2 tbsp olive oil

1 tsp sherry vinegar

1 tsp chilli paste or sauce
    (chipotle works well)

dash of Worcestershire sauce

To serve (optional)

50g halloumi per person

BLACK BEAN, TOMATO & AVOCADO SALAD

There's a great combination of ingredients in this salad, all topped off with a Bloody Mary dressing inspired by that other Mary – the wonderful Mary Berry. No vodka of course, unless you want some! Nice with some grilled halloumi if you fancy it.

Put the red onion in one bowl and the avocado in another. Sprinkle both with salt, then add half the lime juice to each bowl and the lime zest to the avocado bowl. Mix thoroughly and set aside for half an hour.

To make the dressing, put the tomatoes in a small food processor and blitz until smooth. Add the remaining ingredients and process again. Drain the red onion, set the slices aside and add the liquid to the dressing. Taste, then adjust the seasoning.

To assemble, put the leaves in a salad bowl and add the black beans, celery and chopped tomatoes. Add the avocado and the herbs, then pour over half the dressing and mix thoroughly. Sprinkle with the red onion slices and pumpkin seeds, drizzle with the remaining dressing and serve with the halloumi, if using.

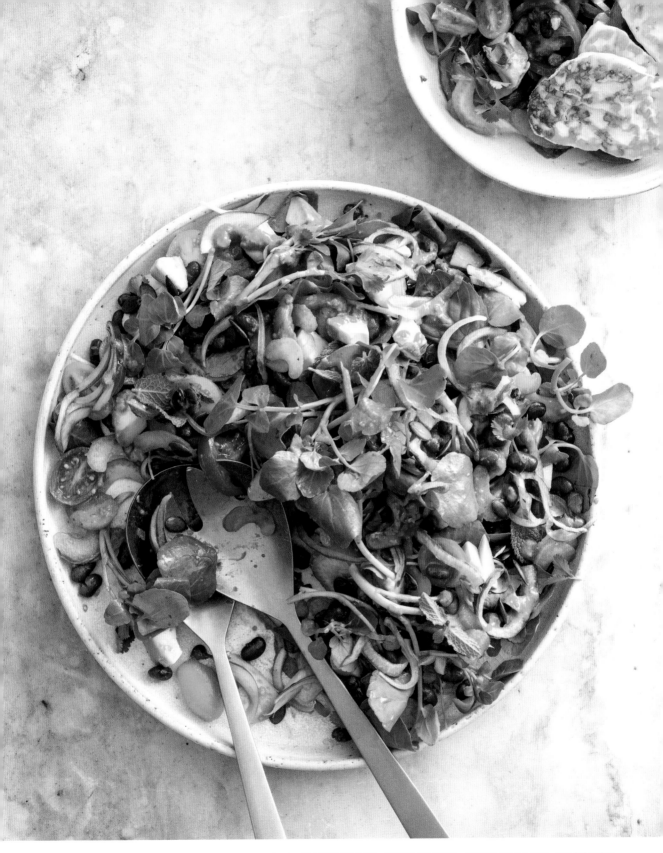

INFO PER SERVING/WITH HALLOUMI: CALORIES 276/448   PROTEIN (G) 9/19   CARBS (G) 18/23   SUGAR (G) 5.5/5/5   FAT (G) 17/30
SATURATED FAT (G) 3/11.5 FIBRE (G) 7/7   SALT (G) 0.2/1.5

oil, for greasing

3 carrots, thinly sliced on the diagonal

200g celeriac, thinly sliced

1 large sweet potato, thinly sliced

200g cauliflower, including leaves and stems, thinly sliced

4 spring onions, finely chopped

2 tbsp finely chopped coriander stems

salt and black pepper

Sauce

400ml can of coconut milk

1 heaped tbsp peanut butter

1 tbsp soy sauce

1 tsp hot sauce

3 garlic cloves, finely crushed

10g root ginger, grated

Topping

50g wholemeal breadcrumbs

1 tbsp sesame seeds

a few coriander sprigs, finely chopped

a few Thai basil leaves, shredded (optional)

2 tsp sesame oil

VEGAN VEGGIE BAKE

Right – this is one of those moments when we get a bit bossy about the method. You do need to slice the vegetables thinly and it's important to layer them up for steaming like we say, as the carrots need the most cooking so have to be closest to the heat. The veg should be cooked until tender but not so much that they break up when mixed into the sauce.

Preheat the oven to 180°C/Fan 160°C/Gas 4. Lightly oil a large ovenproof gratin dish.

Put the vegetables, except the spring onions, into a steamer basket, placing the carrots on the bottom, the celeriac in the middle, followed by the sweet potatoes, then the cauliflower on top. Steam over simmering water until the vegetables are just tender, but firm enough that they won't break up when mixed. This will probably take about 15 minutes, but they might need to cook for a little longer, so check carefully. Remove the veg from the steamer.

Whisk the sauce ingredients together and season with salt and pepper. Put the vegetables in the gratin dish with the spring onions and coriander stems, then season with salt and pepper. Pour over the sauce and mix gently, so everything is thoroughly combined.

For the topping, mix the breadcrumbs with the sesame seeds and herbs. Sprinkle the mixture over the vegetables and then drizzle with sesame oil. Bake in the oven for 25–30 minutes until bubbling and the vegetables are completely tender.

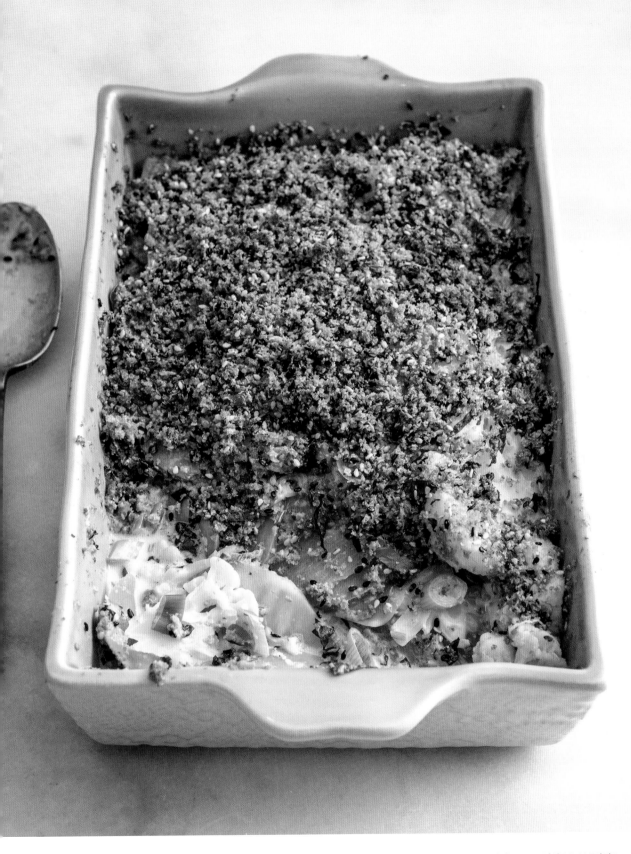

INFO PER SERVING: CALORIES 415 PROTEIN (G) 8 CARBS (G) 37.5 SUGAR (G) 14.5 FAT (G) 24 SATURATED FAT (G) 16 FIBRE (G) 9.5 SALT (G) 1

6–8 red or white chicory, depending on size

2 tbsp olive oil, plus extra for greasing

50ml white wine or vermouth

2 fairly ripe pears, peeled, cored and cut into wedges

leaves from a large thyme sprig

3 slices of Parma ham, pulled into shreds

150ml single cream

1 tbsp crème fraiche

1 tsp plain flour

salt and black pepper

Topping

30g breadcrumbs

30g Gruyère or similar hard cheese, grated

handful of finely chopped parsley leaves

1–2 tsp olive oil

CHICORY & PEAR GRATIN

Chicory or endive – call it what you will, it partners surprisingly well with pears in this simple gratin. We like the ham but you can leave it out if you prefer to keep the dish vegetarian and maybe top the dish with some chopped nuts for protein.

Trim the chicory and cut them into halves or quarters lengthwise, depending on how big they are.

Heat half the olive oil in a large sauté pan. Add half the pieces of chicory and sear them until they are a rich golden brown on the cut sides. Remove them from the pan, add the remaining olive oil and repeat with the remaining chicory.

Put the first batch of chicory back into the pan with the rest and season with salt and pepper. Splash in the wine or vermouth and cover the pan. Leave the chicory to cook over a gentle heat for a few minutes until it's all knife tender through the core.

Preheat the oven to 200°C/Fan 180°C/Gas 6. Transfer the chicory to a lightly oiled ovenproof dish, then toss the pears in the sauté pan over a high heat for just a minute to take on a little colour. Add the pears to the dish with the chicory.

Sprinkle in the thyme and drape the slices of Parma ham over the chicory and pears. Whisk the single cream, crème fraiche and plain flour together and pour the mixture into the dish. Mix the breadcrumbs, cheese and parsley together and sprinkle over the top, then drizzle with the olive oil.

Bake in the oven for about 20 minutes until piping hot, bubbling and golden brown on top. Nice with a simple green salad.

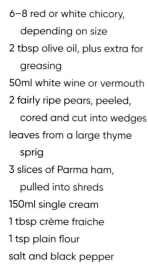

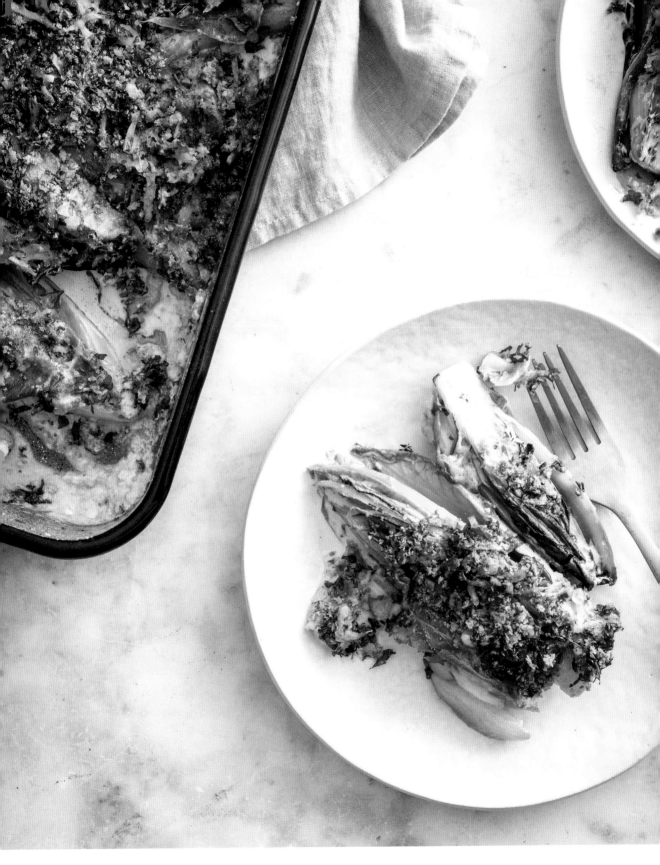

INFO PER SERVING: CALORIES 306 PROTEIN (G) 10 CARBS (G) 17 SUGAR (G) 11 FAT (G) 19 SATURATED FAT (G) 9 FIBRE (G) 7 SALT (G) 0.7

Serves: **4**   Prep: **15 minutes**   Cooking time: **30–35 minutes**

Filling

500g ripe plums, stoned and
   cut into wedges
1 tbsp light brown soft sugar
½ tsp cinnamon

Topping

75g wholemeal flour
60g butter, chilled and diced
50g porridge oats
1 tbsp sesame seeds
1 tbsp sunflower seeds
1 tbsp pumpkin seeds
1 tsp fennel seeds
1 tbsp light brown soft sugar
pinch of salt

PLUM CRUMBLE

There's nothing like a nice fruity crumble to finish off a meal and this one is epic. Having a variety of plant-based foods is important, so this crumble topping with four different types of nutrient-rich seeds really helps towards your total.

Preheat the oven to 180°C/Fan 160°C/Gas 4. Put the plums in an ovenproof dish and sprinkle over the sugar and cinnamon. Mix thoroughly.

For the topping, put the flour into a bowl, add the butter and rub it into the flour. Add the oats, seeds and sugar along with a pinch of salt and stir to combine.

Sprinkle the mixture over the plums in a thin, even layer. Place the dish on a baking tray and bake for 30–35 minutes until the plum juice is bubbling up and the topping is lightly browned. Serve with crème fraiche or custard if you like.

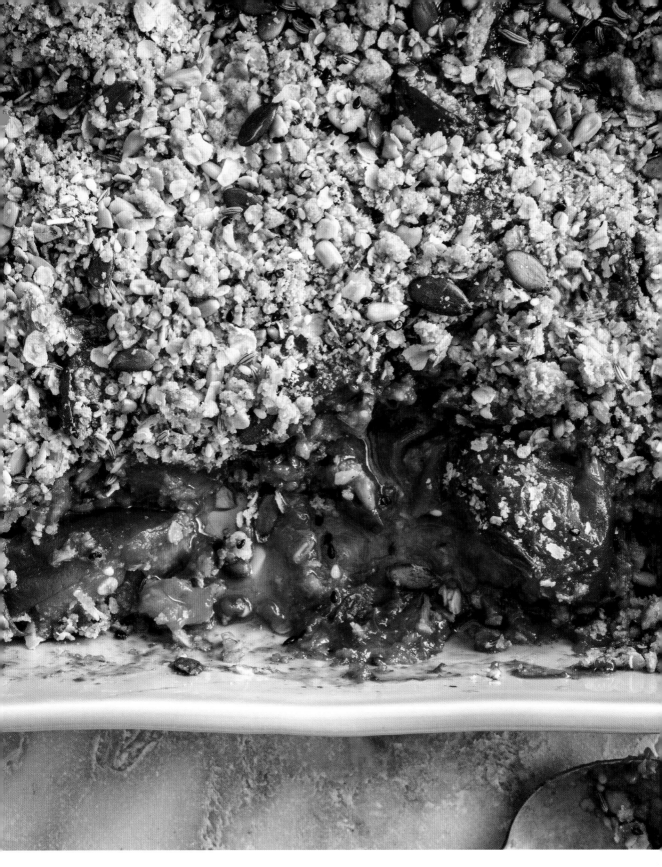

INFO PER SERVING: CALORIES 376   PROTEIN (G) 7.5   CARBS (G) 39   SUGAR (G) 18   FAT (G) 20   SATURATED FAT (G) 9   FIBRE (G) 6.5   SALT (G) 0.5

500g mixed frozen berries

clear apple or grape juice
  (see method)

juice of ½ lemon

1 tbsp honey to taste (optional)

about 4 leaves of gelatine,
  soaked in cold water

250g fresh berries, such as
  blueberries and raspberries

MIXED BERRY JELLY

Frozen berries are generally cheaper than fresh and available all year round, so are ideal for dishes like this jelly. We found four gelatine leaves worked for us, but check the instructions on your packet – it will usually tell you how much you need per amount of liquid. We used apple juice, but you could also make the jelly with diluted cordial if you have some. This is excellent as is and low in calories, so if you really want to push the boat out, you could serve it with a little dollop of ice cream or crème fraiche.

Put the frozen berries in a saucepan and add 150ml of water. Cover the pan and slowly heat so the berries defrost and leach out their liquid. When they have burst and are swimming in juice, strain them through a sieve lined with a piece of muslin or similar. Measure the liquid and make it up to 500ml with the apple or grape juice.

Add the lemon juice and taste, then add a tablespoon of honey if you don't think the mixture is sweet enough. Pour the liquid into a saucepan. Wring out the soaked gelatine leaves and add them to the pan. Stir over a gentle heat until the gelatine has dissolved, then strain the mixture into a jug.

Put the fresh berries into a large bowl or divide them between 4 small bowls and pour the jelly mix over them. Leave to cool to room temperature, stirring regularly to disperse the fruit, then transfer to the fridge to set. Leave for several hours until the jelly has set to a nice wobble.

 Tip: The solids left after straining the berries can be added to a smoothie or mixed with apples to go into a crumble.

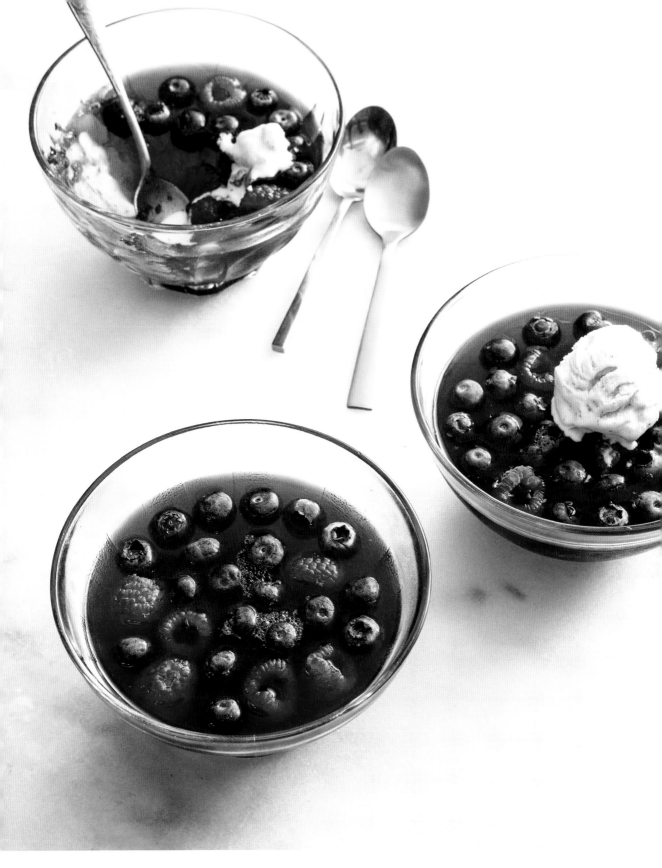

INFO PER SERVING: CALORIES 67 PROTEIN (G) 3 CARBS (G) 11 SUGAR (G) 11 FAT (G) 0 SATURATED FAT (G) 0 FIBRE (G) 4.5 SALT (G) TRACE

FIBRE FEASTS

One of the things we've learned while working on our books is that fibre is hugely important for a healthy gut – and a healthy body. And plenty of fibre can guard against constipation which doesn't help if you're trying to lose weight. Being regular does! Experts say that we should be including about 30 grams of fibre in our diet every day, but most of us don't manage that. Good sources of fibre include vegetables and fruit (particularly with the skin on), as well as whole grains, brown rice, nuts, seeds and pulses. And all these foods help you feel fuller for longer and so you're less likely to reach for fast-food snacks. Be careful, though. Suddenly increasing your fibre intake if you're not used to it can make you feel bloated, so take it gently at first and your digestive system will soon adapt.

75g chia seeds

2 tbsp maple syrup

2 tbsp yoghurt or kefir

250ml milk

pinch of cinnamon

a few drops of vanilla extract

Topping

2 tbsp oats

1 tbsp flaked almonds

a generous pinch of cinnamon

pinch of salt

1 tbsp maple syrup

a few mint sprigs

Fruit

200g blueberries

4 kiwi fruits, peeled and sliced

juice of 1 lime

a few mint leaves, shredded

CHIA SEED PUDDINGS

Chia seeds have become hugely popular because they're so rich in fibre. Just one of these little puds contains ten grams of fibre – a third of your ideal total for the day. The yoghurt in the mix helps to soften the seeds, making them easier to digest. The puddings are really easy to prepare at the end of the day, ready to finish off the next morning and enjoy for breakfast.

Start the night before you intend on eating the puddings. Put the chia seeds in a container and add the syrup, yoghurt or kefir, milk, cinnamon and vanilla. Stir, then cover and leave in the fridge overnight. The seeds will swell up and absorb the liquid.

For the topping, put the oats, almonds and cinnamon in a dry frying pan with a pinch of salt. Stir until everything smells lightly toasted, then drizzle over the maple syrup. Continue to stir until the maple syrup coats the oats and nuts, then set aside to cool.

When you're ready to eat, divide two-thirds of the blueberries between 4 glasses. Top with some of the chia seed mixture. Toss the kiwi fruits with the lime juice and shredded mint leaves and add to the glasses, then spoon over the rest of the chia mixture. Sprinkle with the topping and the remaining blueberries and add sprigs of mint. Serve immediately.

 Tip: These are great for breakfast, but kiwi fruits are believed to aid a restful night's sleep, so you might want to try this combo at bedtime too.

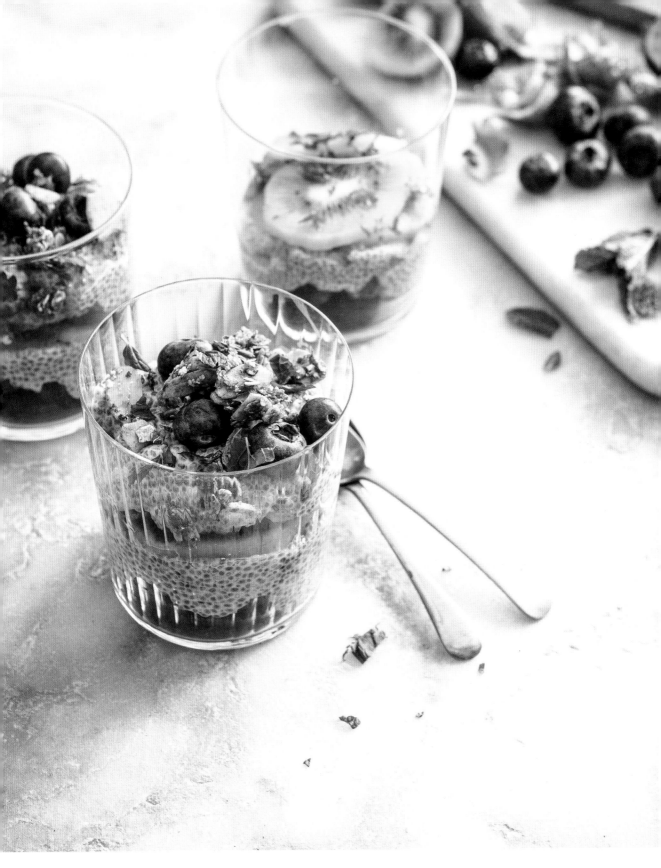

INFO PER SERVING: CALORIES 300 PROTEIN (G) 8.5 CARBS (G) 36 SUGAR (G) 22.5 FAT (G) 11.5 SATURATED FAT (G) 2.5 FIBRE (G) 10 SALT (G) 0.4

4 large or 8 small potatoes

400g broccoli florets

1 tbsp olive oil

1 small onion, finely chopped

100g black pudding or chorizo, diced

1 garlic clove, finely chopped

½ tsp mixed dried herbs

50g Cheddar or other hard cheese, grated

salt and black pepper

STUFFED POTATO SKINS

If you're worried about heating up the oven just for baking some potatoes, we've given you some other options, so take your pick. As long as you end up with crispy fibre-rich skins to pack with the tasty filling, that's what counts.

If baking the potatoes in the oven, preheat the oven to 200°C/Fan 180°C/Gas 6. Pierce the potatoes all over with a skewer, then put them on a baking tray and bake them for 1–1½ hours, depending on size.

Alternatively, you can microwave them. Pierce the potatoes in the same way, then cook in the microwave for 4 minutes. Turn them over and cook for a further 4 minutes and then keep cooking at 1-minute bursts until completely cooked – again, this will depend on size. You can also pressure cook your potatoes – pierce them as above and put them in the steamer basket with 2cm of water in the base. Cook for 15–20 minutes at high pressure, depending on size, then allow the pressure to drop naturally.

Prepare the filling. Steam the broccoli florets until tender, then chop them roughly. Heat the oil in a frying pan and add the onion. Sauté until translucent, then turn up the heat and add the black pudding or chorizo. When well browned, add the garlic and herbs and stir for a further minute. Stir in the broccoli florets and season.

When the potatoes are cool enough to handle, cut them in half and scoop out most of the flesh, leaving a 1cm thick border. (Use the scooped out potato to make hash, mash or fish cakes, or add it to bread dough.)

Preheat the oven to 200°C/Fan 180°C/Gas 6 if you have baked your potatoes by a non-oven method. Arrange the potato skins on a baking tray and fill them with the broccoli mixture. Sprinkle over the cheese and bake in the oven for about 15 minutes until the cheese has melted and browned.

 Tip: If you prefer to go veggie, just leave out the black pudding or chorizo – or try the vegetarian version of black pudding. We think it's good.

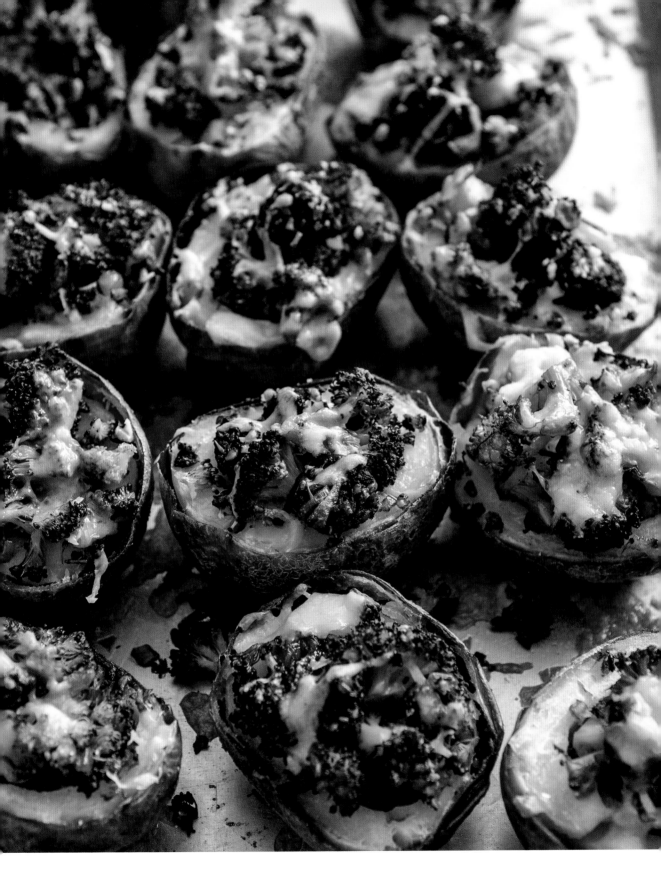

CALORIES 365 PROTEIN (G) 15 CARBS (G) 42 SUGAR (G) 6 FAT (G) 13 SATURATED FAT (G) 5.5 FIBRE (G) 9 SALT (G) 0.8

500g carrots, cut into batons
1 tbsp olive oil
1 red onion, finely sliced

Salad

250g green beans
150g cooked bulgur wheat
    (about 50g uncooked
    weight)
75g radishes, finely sliced
25g dates, pitted and finely
    chopped
25g pumpkin seeds
salt and black pepper

Dressing

1 tbsp tahini
1 tbsp olive oil
juice of 1 lemon
½ tsp honey
generous pinch of chilli flakes

Garnish

a few mint leaves
a few parsley leaves
1 tsp za'atar (optional)
1 tsp sumac

ROAST CARROT & GREEN BEAN SALAD

Something magical happens to carrots when they're roasted – the flavour intensifies, making this salad something special. Plenty of other fibre-rich ingredients turn this into a real feast and the little pumpkin seeds also provide valuable magnesium and zinc.

Preheat the oven to 200°C/Fan 180°C/Gas 6. Put the carrots in a bowl and drizzle them with the olive oil. Toss to thoroughly combine, then place in a roasting tin and roast for 20 minutes.

Drop the red onion slices into the same bowl and give them a stir – they will pick up the residue of oil. Sprinkle the onion over the carrots, put the tin back in the oven and roast for another 10–15 minutes until the carrots are tender and the onion is crisp. Remove them from the oven and leave to cool to room temperature.

Bring a pan of water to the boil, add the green beans and bring back to the boil. Drain and refresh in cold water, then set aside.

To make the dressing, whisk everything together and season with salt and pepper. Thin it with a little water if necessary.

To assemble, sprinkle half the bulgur wheat over a platter, then arrange the carrots, onions and beans over the top. Sprinkle with the remaining bulgur wheat, then top with the radishes, dates and pumpkin seeds.

Drizzle over the dressing, then garnish with the herbs, a sprinkling of za'atar, if using, and the sumac.

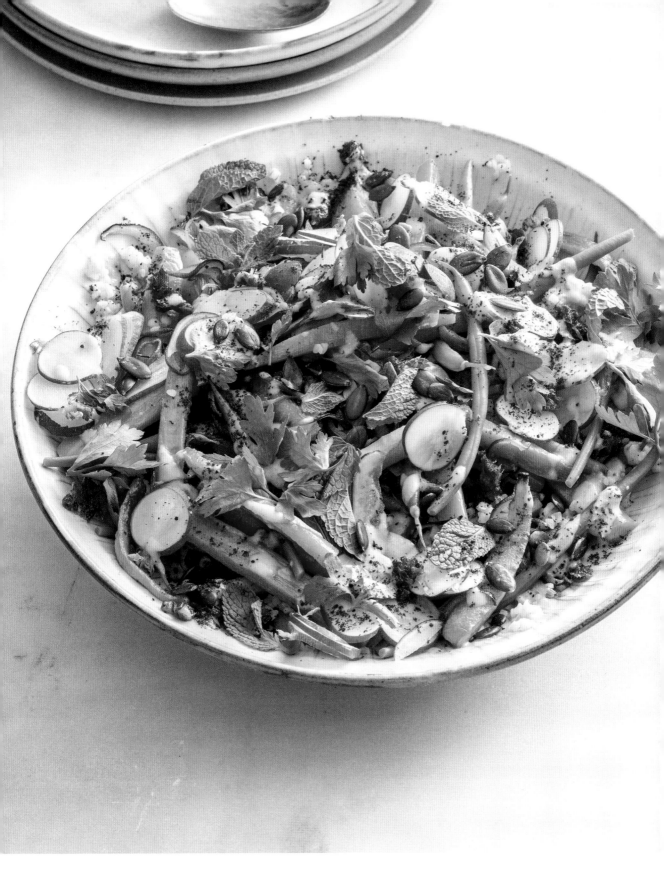

BEETROOT, GOAT'S CHEESE & ORZO SALAD

50g orzo

200g broad beans
(frozen are fine)

150g salad leaves, such
as rocket or watercress

250g cooked beetroot,
cut into chunks

150g soft goat's cheese,
broken up or sliced

50g hazelnuts

salt and black pepper

Dressing

1 tbsp olive oil

2 tsp red wine vinegar
or sherry vinegar

juice of ½ lemon

½ tsp honey

½ tsp dried mint

1 small shallot, finely sliced

Gremolata

zest of 1 lemon, finely chopped

1 garlic clove, very finely
chopped

small bunch of dill, finely
chopped

leaves from 2 mint sprigs,
finely chopped (optional)

We sometimes skin broad beans to reveal their bright green prettiness, but we suggest leaving the skins on for this vibrant salad to increase the fibre content. Saves time too. Beetroot and goat's cheese are great partners and, if you like, you could use puy lentils instead of orzo to up the fibre content even more.

First cook the orzo. Bring a saucepan of water to the boil and add plenty of salt. Add the orzo and cook for 3–4 minutes until almost cooked, then add the broad beans. Drain and leave to cool to room temperature.

To make the dressing, whisk the olive oil, vinegar, lemon juice, honey and dried mint together. Season with salt and pepper and stir in the shallot.

To make the gremolata, mix the lemon zest, garlic and herbs together.

To assemble, put the salad leaves in a serving bowl or platter and add the beetroot, the cooled orzo and broad beans. Toss in the dressing, then top with the goat's cheese and hazelnuts. Sprinkle with the gremolata and serve.

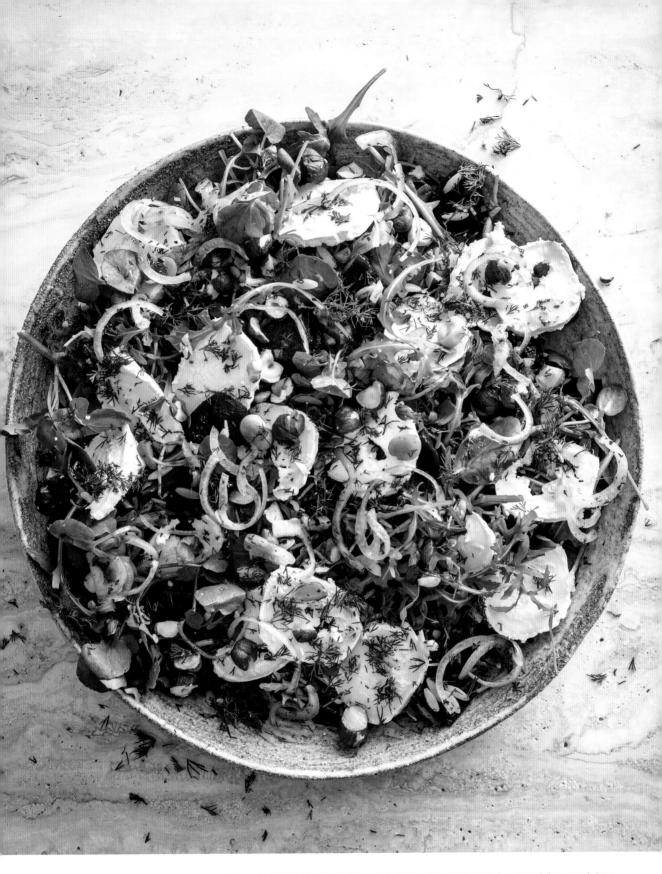

INFO PER SERVING: CALORIES 353   PROTEIN (G) 16   CARBS (G) 21   SUGAR (G) 8   FAT (G) 21   SATURATED FAT (G) 8   FIBRE (G) 8   SALT (G) 0.7

MEATLESS MEATLOAF

1 large carrot, coarsely grated

1 large courgette, coarsely grated

1 tbsp olive oil

1 onion, very finely chopped

1 celery stick, very finely chopped

2 garlic cloves, finely chopped

zest of 1 lemon

1 rosemary sprig, finely chopped

a few parsley sprigs, finely chopped

1 tsp dried oregano

200g cooked lentils (make sure they're not too mushy)

75g wholemeal breadcrumbs

100g halloumi, coarsely grated

4 tbsp seeds (mix of sesame, sunflower, pumpkin and chia)

2 tbsp tomato purée

1 egg

salt and black pepper

No meat in this, but there are lots of fibre-rich goodies to delight you. Good served hot with tomato sauce and green veg or cold with a salad, the meatloaf has a nice moist texture and lots of flavour. Just make sure that the lentils aren't too wet or they will make the mixture too claggy in the centre.

Put the carrot and courgette into a colander and sprinkle with a teaspoon of salt. Leave to stand for at least half an hour – you should find that they have collapsed down a little. Squeeze out as much liquid as you can.

Heat the oil in a frying pan and add the onion and celery. Fry until translucent, then add the grated carrot and courgette. Continue to sauté until they take on a little colour, then add the garlic, lemon zest and herbs. Stir for another couple of minutes, then tip everything into a bowl. Add all the remaining ingredients and season with plenty of pepper. Taste a little of the mixture for salt – you may not need to add any because the vegetables and halloumi will add quite a bit. Mix thoroughly.

Preheat the oven to 180°C/Fan 160°C/Gas 4 and line a small loaf tin with baking parchment. Press the mixture into the tin and cover with lightly oiled parchment or foil. Place in the oven and bake for about half an hour, then uncover and cook for a further 15–20 minutes until the loaf is piping hot with a lightly browned crust.

Leave to stand for a few minutes before turning out and slicing. Nice with a tomato sauce (see page 184).

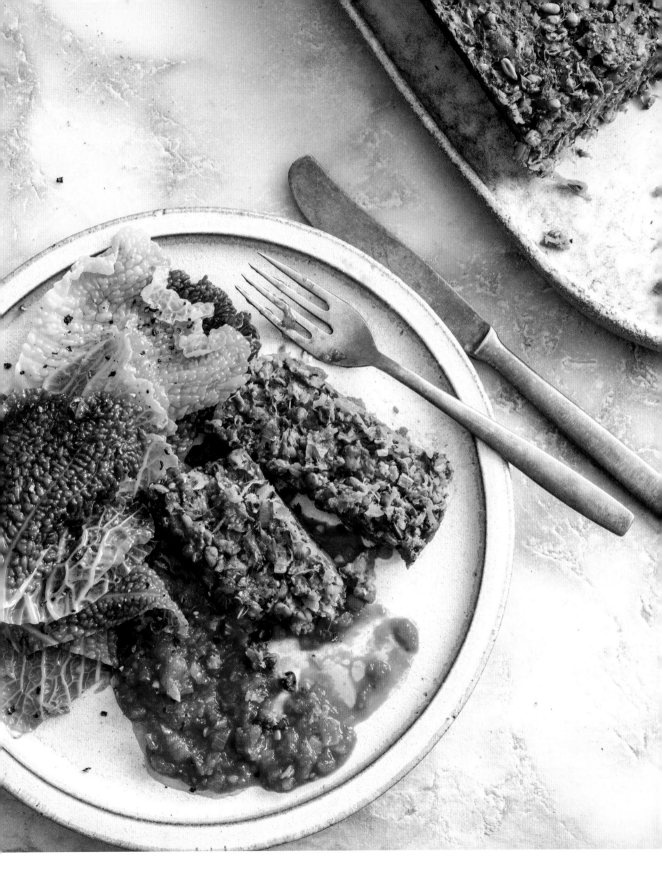

INFO PER SERVING (MEATLOAF): CALORIES 362 PROTEIN (G) 20 CARBS (G) 25 SUGAR (G) 7 FAT (G) 18 SATURATED FAT (G) 6 FIBRE (G) 9 SALT (G) 1.1

1 tbsp olive oil

1 large onion, finely chopped

1 large aubergine, diced

3 garlic cloves, finely chopped

1 fresh red chilli, finely chopped
    (or ½ tsp chilli powder)

1 tsp dried oregano

100ml white wine

400g can of tomatoes or fresh
    equivalent

400g can of chickpeas,
    drained

basil sprig and a few torn basil
    leaves

zest of ½ lemon

400g spaghetti or linguine

salt and black pepper

To serve

Parmesan, grated

PASTA WITH AUBERGINES & CHICKPEAS

Aubergines can really soak up oil, but for this recipe we've kept the oil to a minimum. Both aubergines and chickpeas are classic pasta partners so we decided to bring them together in this dish, which is packed with texture and flavour as well as fibre.

Heat the oil in a saucepan and add the onion. Cook for 5 minutes over a medium heat, then add the aubergine and continue to cook for a further 5 minutes, stirring regularly. Add the garlic and chilli and cook for another minute.

Sprinkle in the oregano and season with salt and pepper, then turn up the heat and add the white wine. Allow it to boil for a couple of minutes, then add the tomatoes, swilling out the can with 200ml of water. Add the chickpeas to the sauce and bring to the boil.

Cover the pan, turn down the heat and simmer for about 20 minutes. Add a sprig of basil, then continue to cook, uncovered, for a further 10 minutes, stirring regularly. Stir in the lemon zest.

Meanwhile, cook the pasta in plenty of salted, boiling water and drain. Remove the basil sprig from the sauce. Ladle the sauce over the pasta and add a few torn basil leaves and serve with some grated Parmesan.

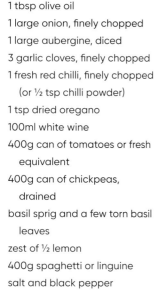

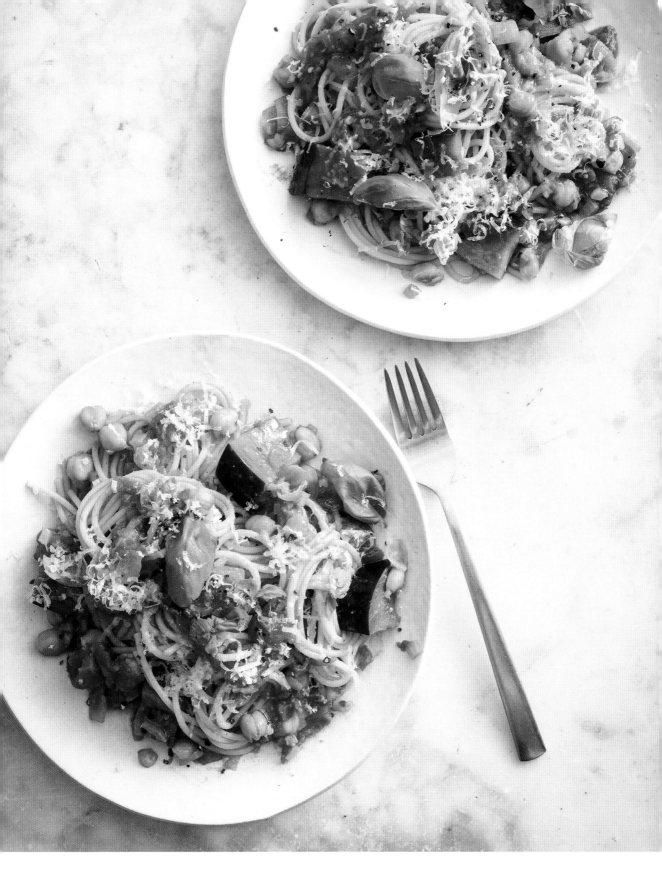

INFO PER SERVING: CALORIES 544 PROTEIN (G) 19.4 CARBS (G) 91 SUGAR (G) 10.4 FAT (G) 6.5 SATURATED FAT (G) 1 FIBRE (G) 12.5 SALT (G) 0.1

1 tbsp olive oil

300g lamb mince

1 onion, finely chopped

1 large carrot, coarsely grated

4 garlic cloves, finely chopped

10g root ginger, grated

2 tbsp curry powder (strength up to you)

200g chopped tomatoes

300g frozen peas

6 cubes of frozen spinach

300ml chicken, vegetable or lamb stock or water

400g cooked brown basmati rice (175–200g uncooked)

juice of 1 lemon

salt and black pepper

To serve

small bunch of coriander, finely chopped

3–4 green chillies, finely sliced

KEEMA BIRYANI

This ticks all the boxes in terms of health: cooked and cooled rice, plenty of veg and some citrus juice to help your body absorb the iron from the vegetables. It's an easy way to make a biryani to be proud of and it's dead tasty to eat.

Heat a teaspoon of the oil in a large frying pan, add the lamb mince and sear it on all sides. Break it up with a wooden spoon and continue to fry until it's just cooked through and has rendered out plenty of fat. Remove the lamb from the pan with a slotted spoon and drain it on kitchen paper. Discard the fat.

Heat the remaining oil in a large saucepan. Add the onion and carrot and sauté until the onion is soft and translucent, then add the garlic and ginger. Cook for another couple of minutes, then stir in the curry powder. Add the browned lamb to the saucepan and stir to combine.

Add the tomatoes, peas and spinach (fine to add from frozen) and pour the stock or water into the pan. Season with salt and pepper, then bring to the boil, turn down the heat and cover the pan. Leave to simmer for about 15 minutes, then remove the lid and continue to simmer until the sauce has reduced and thickened.

Add the cooked rice to the pan and gently fold it in to combine. Make sure the rice is completely heated through, then add the lemon juice. Sprinkle with plenty of coriander and green chillies before serving.

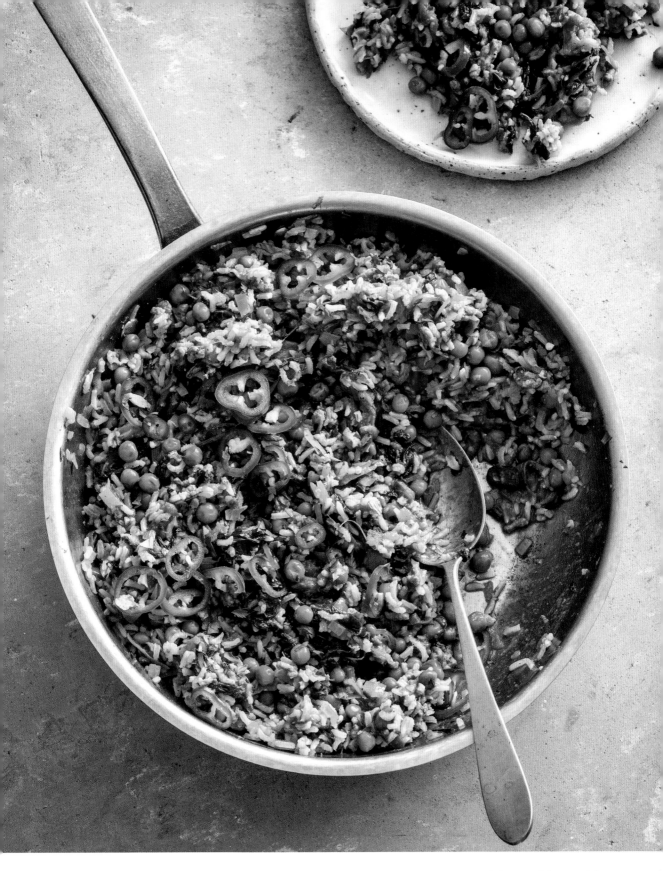

INFO PER SERVING: CALORIES 461 PROTEIN (G) 27 CARBS (G) 46 SUGAR (G) 9 FAT (G) 16.5 SATURATED FAT (G) 6 FIBRE (G) 11 SALT (G) 0.5

1 tbsp olive oil

1 large onion, diced

3 celery sticks, diced

1 green pepper, diced

1 sweet potato, diced (or
  equivalent in squash)

200g cavolo nero, shredded

3 garlic cloves, finely chopped

1 tbsp Cajun spice mix (shop-
  bought or see p.185)

1 tsp dried thyme

800ml vegetable stock

400g can of beans (pinto/red
  kidney/black)

400g can of chopped
  tomatoes

salt and black pepper

Dumplings

150g self-raising flour

125g fine cornmeal

50g butter, chilled and diced

100ml buttermilk

1 egg

Garnishes (optional)

grated cheese

pickled chillies

BEAN & SWEET POTATO STEW WITH CORNMEAL DUMPLINGS

With sweet potato and cornmeal, this fibre-rich recipe was inspired by our travels in the southern USA. The light fluffy dumplings are perfect partners for the veg stew and they soak up the tasty juices beautifully.

Heat the olive oil in a large saucepan or a flameproof casserole dish. Add the onion, celery and pepper and sauté until the onion and celery look translucent. Add the sweet potato or squash, cavolo nero, garlic, spices and thyme, and stir to combine.

Pour in the stock, beans and tomatoes and season with salt and pepper. Bring to the boil, then cover the pan and simmer for about 20 minutes.

For the dumplings, put the flour and cornmeal in a bowl and season with salt and pepper. Add the butter and rub it into the flour and cornmeal. Beat the buttermilk and egg together and mix with the dry ingredients – you will end up with quite a firm dough. Roll the mixture into 8 balls and drop them on top of the stew.

Simmer for a further 15–20 minutes, covered, until the dumplings are risen and glossy and the vegetables are tender. Serve with the garnishes, if using.

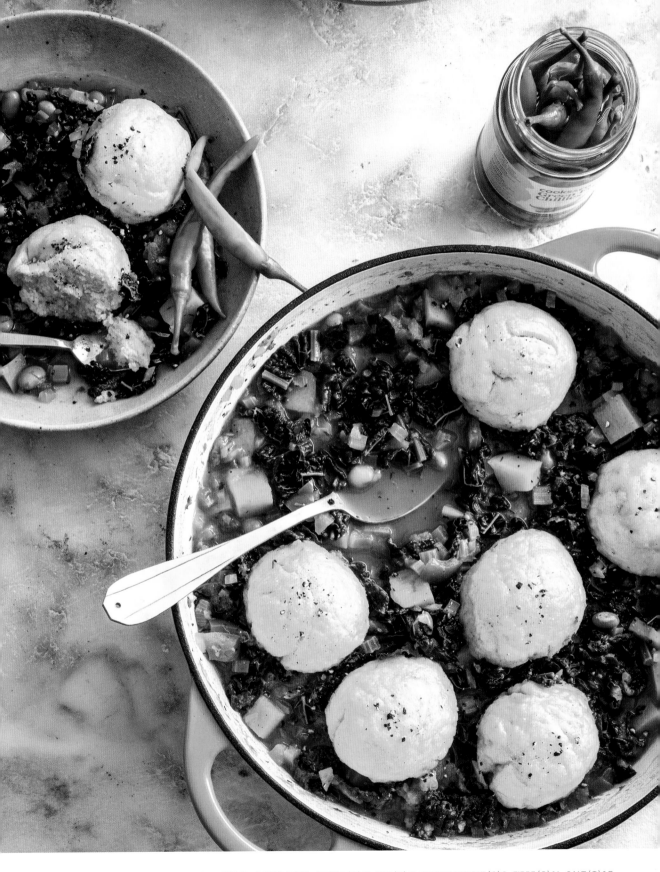

INFO PER SERVING: CALORIES 615 PROTEIN (G) 19 CARBS (G) 85 SUGAR (G) 15 FAT (G) 19 SATURATED FAT (G) 8 FIBRE (G) 16 SALT (G) 1.7

1 x 1.2–1.5kg chicken

2 tbsp olive oil

2 tarragon sprigs

1 garlic bulb, cloves left
    unpeeled, but pierced
    with a knife point

2 onions, cut into wedges

2 celery sticks, cut into chunks

4 carrots, cut into chunks

10g dried mushrooms
    (no need to soak)

150g pearl barley

600ml chicken or vegetable
    stock

2 tbsp finely chopped parsley,
    to garnish

salt and black pepper

To serve

lightly steamed greens

POT-ROAST CHICKEN WITH BARLEY

Roast chicken is a treat we never tire of and here we pot-roast it with some barley for a fibre-rich version of a Sunday dinner. Pearl barley is good or you could use wholegrain barley for extra fibre – it will need to cook for longer, though. And you can add extra root veg, such as parsnips, if you fancy.

Preheat the oven to 170°C/Fan 150°C/Gas 3½. Rub the chicken all over with half the olive oil, then sprinkle with salt and pepper. Tuck one of the tarragon sprigs inside the cavity, along with a few of the garlic cloves.

Heat the remaining oil in a large flameproof casserole dish. Add the onions, celery and carrots and sauté over a high heat for several minutes until they start to brown. Crumble in the dried mushrooms. Finely chop the leaves from the remaining sprig of tarragon and stir them in, along with the remaining garlic cloves. Stir in the barley and pour over the stock, then season with salt and pepper.

Bring to the boil, then add the chicken to the dish. Cover with a lid, place in the oven and cook for an hour.

After an hour, remove the lid – the barley should be just cooked through and the chicken should be almost ready too. Turn the oven up to 200°C/Fan 180°C/Gas 6 and cook for another 15–20 minutes until the chicken has browned and is completely cooked through.

Remove the chicken from the dish, cover it lightly with some foil and leave it to rest for 10–15 minutes. For a creamier finish, remove the garlic cloves from the pot, squeeze out the flesh and stir it into the barley and vegetables. Alternatively, leave the garlic cloves as they are for everyone to squeeze out at the table. Garnish with parsley and serve with greens on the side.

Tip: If you don't have a casserole dish that's large enough, use a roasting tin and cover the chicken tightly with a double layer of foil. You might need a little extra liquid, as the barley will be more spaced out and the liquid will evaporate more quickly.

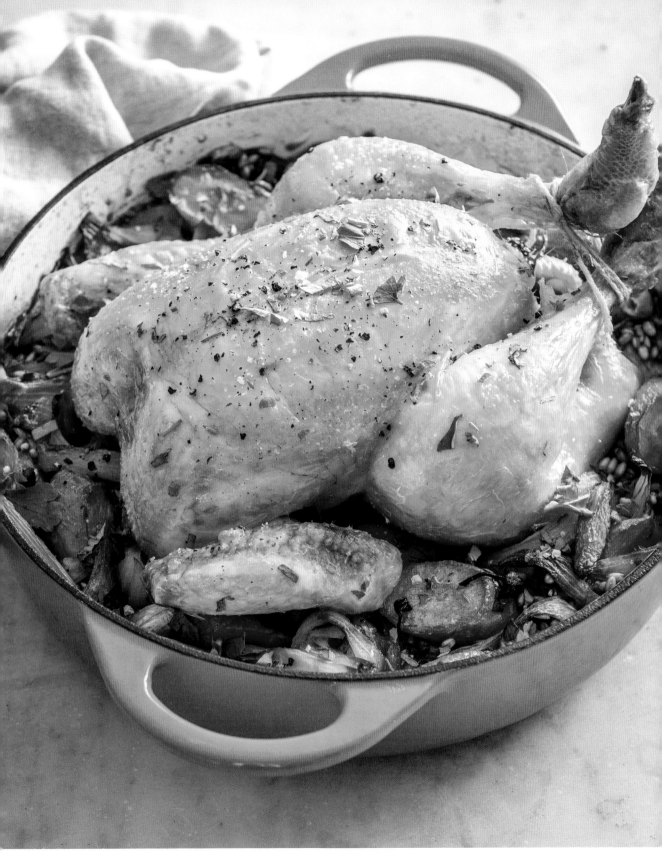

INFO PER SERVING: CALORIES 525 PROTEIN (G) 49 CARBS (G) 45 SUGAR (G) 11.5 FAT (G) 14 SATURATED FAT (G) 3 FIBRE (G) 11 SALT (G) 0.7

3 tbsp olive oil

500g lean stewing lamb, diced

1 red onion, thickly sliced

250g carrots, sliced

3 garlic cloves, finely chopped

1 tbsp tagine spice mix (see p.185) or ras-el-hanout

pinch of saffron, soaked in a little warm water (optional)

needles from 1 rosemary sprig, finely chopped

500ml chicken or vegetable stock or water

400g can of chickpeas, drained

12 pitted prunes

1 small red or green pointed cabbage, cut into wedges

juice of ½ lemon

small bunch of parsley, finely chopped

salt and black pepper

To serve

wholemeal couscous (optional)

LAMB & CHICKPEA TAGINE

Chickpeas, cabbage and prunes with the tasty lamb make this a real festival of fibre. A special treat your family and friends will love.

Heat a tablespoon of the oil in a large flameproof casserole dish. When it's hot, add the lamb and sear it on all sides. Remove the lamb from the pan and set it aside.

Add another tablespoon of oil and sauté the red onion and carrots over a high heat for 5 minutes. Add the garlic and cook for a further 2 minutes, then put the lamb back in the casserole dish. Stir in the spice mix or ras-el-hanout, the saffron, if using, and the rosemary, then pour in just enough of the stock or water to cover the meat. Season with salt and pepper, then bring to the boil.

Cover the pan and turn down the heat. Simmer for 45 minutes until the lamb is well on the way to being tender, then add the chickpeas and prunes.

Heat the remaining oil in a large frying pan. Sear the cabbage wedges on the cut sides, then add them to the casserole dish. Simmer the tagine for a further 30–45 minutes, until the cabbage and meat are completely tender. Add the lemon juice, then sprinkle with the parsley. Serve with wholemeal couscous for extra fibre.

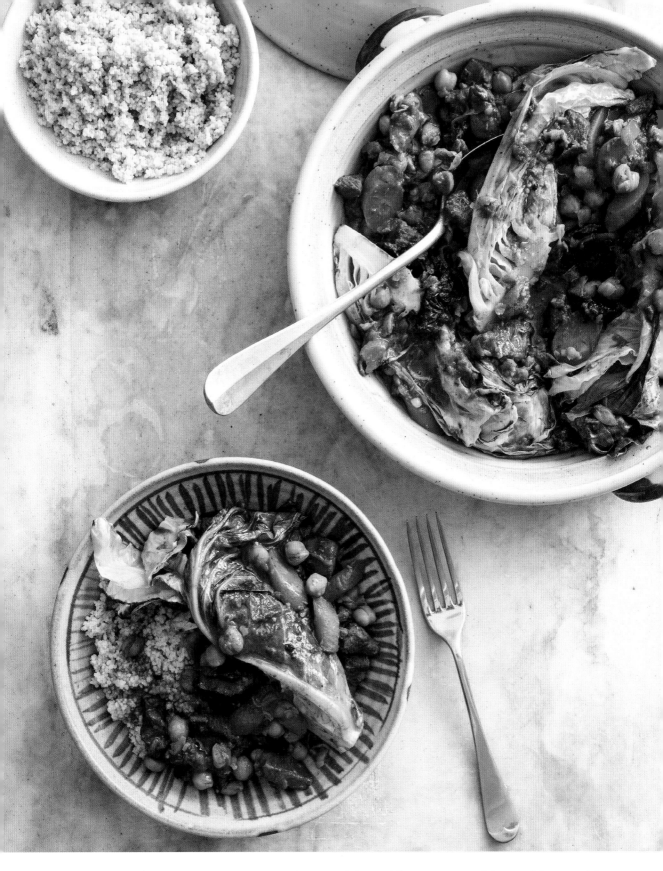

INFO PER SERVING: CALORIES 479 PROTEIN (G) 37 CARBS (G) 30 SUGAR (G) 19 FAT (G) 21 SATURATED FAT (G) 6 FIBRE (G) 12.5 SALT (G) 0.5

100g brown basmati rice

pinch of salt

up to 750ml whole milk

1 small can (104ml) of
    evaporated milk

½ tsp ground cinnamon

½ tsp vanilla extract

50ml maple syrup

1 apple, cored and coarsely
    grated

25g raisins or sultanas

50g pitted prunes or dates,
    chopped

To serve

drizzle of maple syrup

200g raspberries

BROWN RICE PUDDING

Our mams used to use white pudding rice, but we've tried upping the fibre content of one of our favourite puds by using brown – and we like it. Adding some dried fruit, such as prunes and dates, brings more fibre and some nice extra sweetness. And would you believe that the little raspberry is high in fibre as well as vitamin C.

Put the brown rice in a saucepan with a pinch of salt and add 300ml of water. Cover and bring to the boil, then turn down the heat and leave the rice to simmer for about half an hour until all the water has been absorbed. At this stage the rice will be cooked, but with a firmer texture than you want for rice pudding. Remove the saucepan from the heat and leave to stand for at least 10 minutes – the rice will continue to steam.

Add 500ml of the milk, the evaporated milk, cinnamon, vanilla extract, maple syrup, apple, raisins or sultanas and prunes or dates. Bring to the boil, then turn the heat down and cook, uncovered, for at least half an hour until most of the milk has been absorbed by the rice and the apple has broken down. Keep stirring regularly.

Taste for texture and sweetness – the rice should have softened and given out a lot of starch to thicken the liquid around it. If it needs longer, add the remaining milk and continue to cook until you have the right texture – this might take up to an hour in total, so be patient! The rice is ready when the texture is as soft as you would expect from white pudding rice.

Serve with an extra drizzle of maple syrup and some fresh raspberries.

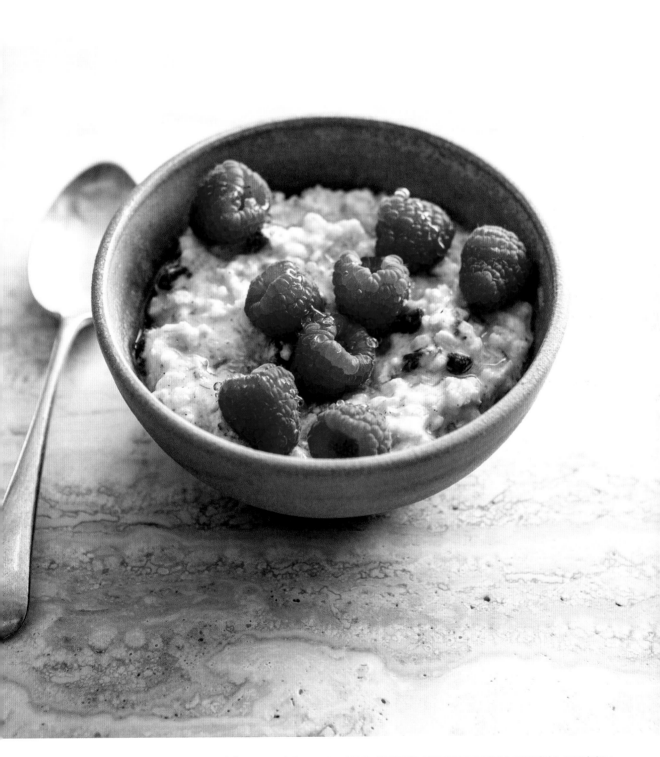

INFO PER SERVING: CALORIES 361 PROTEIN (G) 12 CARBS (G) 55 SUGAR (G) 34 FAT (G) 10 SATURATED FAT (G) 6 FIBRE (G) 4 SALT (G) 0.6

oil, for greasing

300g wholemeal bread, diced (preferably sourdough)

25g plain flour (white or wholemeal)

1 tsp baking powder

100g light brown soft sugar

25g pecan nuts, very finely chopped

1 tsp ground cinnamon

pinch of salt

100g raisins

100ml strong tea or marsala

300ml milk

2 eggs

50g butter, melted

1 tsp vanilla extract

400g can of peaches in juice or water, drained and diced

To serve

2 tsp granulated sugar

½ tsp ground cinnamon

PEACH & RAISIN BREAD PUDDING

If you have any stale bread, do yourself a big favour and use it to make this scrumptious pud. Enjoy it hot with custard or cut it into squares and serve as a cake for tea time. If possible, plan ahead for this one because ideally the mixture needs soaking for a couple of hours before baking.

Grease a 20cm square baking tin or similar-sized ovenproof dish with a little oil. If your tin is loose-bottomed, line it with some foil and baking parchment or the pudding will leak.

Put the bread, flour, baking powder, sugar, pecans and cinnamon in a large bowl with a pinch of salt and mix thoroughly. Put the raisins in a small saucepan and cover with the tea or marsala. Bring to the boil, then leave to simmer until virtually all of the liquid has been absorbed by the raisins. Remove from the heat.

Whisk the milk, eggs, melted butter and vanilla extract together. Pour this over the bread mixture and mix thoroughly, breaking up the bread as much as possible – we find the simplest way to do this is with our hands. Stir in the raisins and peaches, then leave to stand for at least a couple of hours or, even better, overnight.

When you are ready to bake your pudding, preheat the oven to 180°C/Fan 160°C/Gas 4. Transfer the mixture to the baking tin or dish and press it down as much as possible, trying to make sure that any raisins are pushed well into the mixture.

Bake for about 1–1½ hours, checking regularly to make sure the top isn't browning too much – cover it with a single layer of foil if it is. When done, the pudding should feel springy to the touch and not too soft and should be a rich golden brown. Remove from the oven and turn out.

To serve, mix the granulated sugar with the cinnamon and sprinkle over the cake. Cut into squares and serve hot for pudding or leave it to cool down and eat as a cake. It will keep in an airtight container for a week.

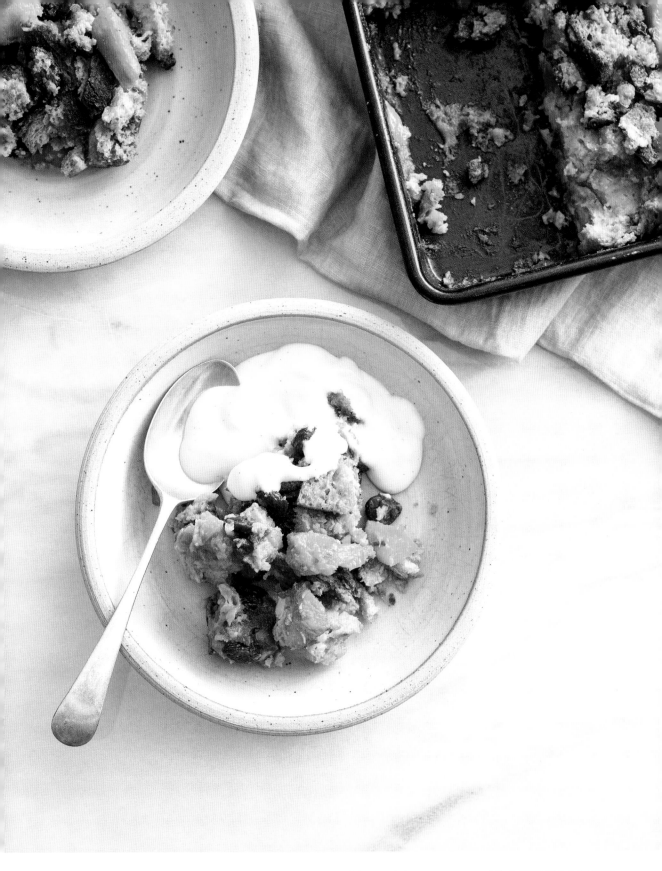

INFO PER SERVING: CALORIES 424 PROTEIN (G) 11 CARBS (G) 59 SUGAR (G) 37 FAT (G) 15 SATURATED FAT (G) 6.5 FIBRE (G) 5 SALT (G) 1.2

BRAIN FOOD

We're really pleased to learn that eating well can even help the brain and memory which is fantastic news! Research shows that a diet of good fresh foods rich in vitamins, minerals and antioxidants can nourish your brain and help to protect it from damage and decline as you get older. Did you know that 60 per cent of the brain is fat and so it needs essential fatty acids, particularly omega-3, for good function? Oily fish is great for the brain and memory, as are berries, such as blueberries, leafy greens, peppers, nuts and seeds. Spices such as turmeric and ginger are also thought to aid brain function and you'll find a recipe for a delicious ginger and turmeric tea in this chapter.

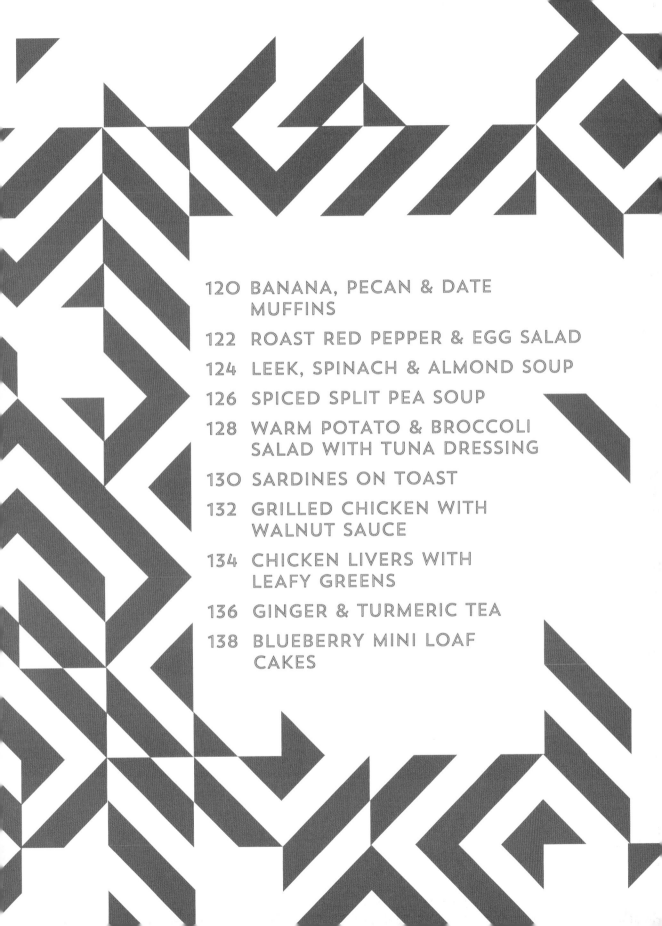

50ml oil (olive, sunflower
   or rapeseed), plus extra
   for greasing
3 ripe bananas, mashed
75ml maple syrup
100ml yoghurt or soured cream
1 egg
1 tsp vanilla extract
225g wholemeal or plain flour
1 tsp bicarbonate of soda
1 tsp cinnamon
rasp of nutmeg
pinch of salt
75g pecans or walnuts,
   finely chopped
50g soft dates, pitted and
   finely chopped

BANANA, PECAN & DATE MUFFINS

Some studies have shown that nuts are really good for your brain, so that's a great reason to treat yourself to these scrumptious little muffins. Nothing like a warm muffin straight from the oven to cheer you up in the morning.

Preheat the oven to 180°C/Fan 160°C/Gas 4. Line a 12-hole muffin tin with muffin cases or lightly oil the tin.

Mix the oil, mashed bananas, syrup, yoghurt or soured cream, egg and vanilla in a large bowl. Mix the flour, bicarb, spices, a generous pinch of salt and 50g of the nuts in another bowl. Stir in the dates, making sure they don't clump together – they may well do if they are very sticky, but the flour will help separate them.

Add the dry ingredients to the wet and fold them together, keeping the mixing to an absolute minimum – don't worry if there's still the odd streak of flour.

Spoon the mixture into the muffin cases – they will be almost full – and sprinkle with the remaining nuts. Bake the muffins in the oven for about 20 minutes until well risen, springy to touch and lightly golden, then leave them to cool in the tin. Enjoy the muffins while they're still warm, but they will keep for up to a week in an airtight tin.

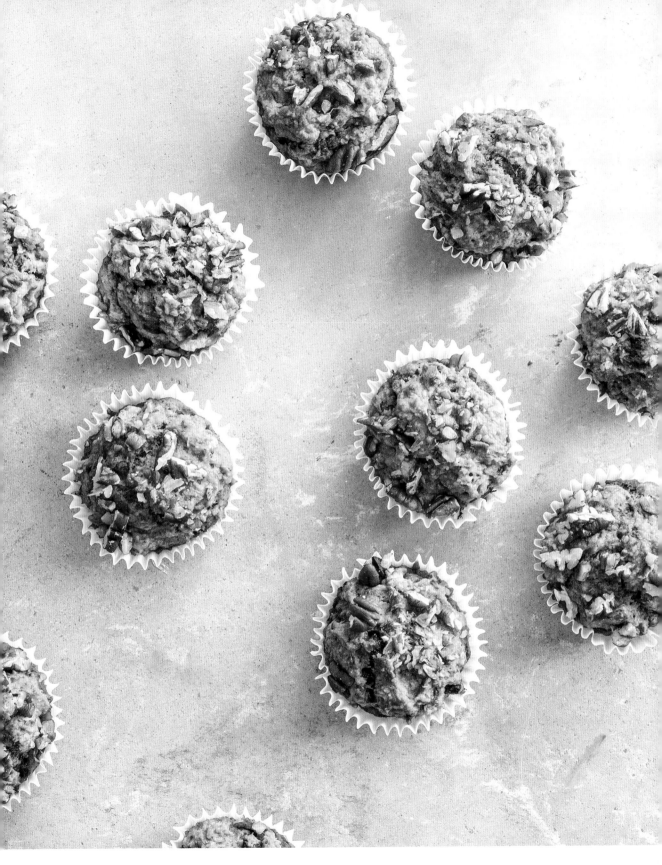

INFO PER MUFFIN: CALORIES 181   PROTEIN (G) 3   CARBS (G) 23   SUGAR (G) 10   FAT (G) 8   SATURATED FAT (G) 1   FIBRE (G) 3   SALT (G) 0.3

1 red onion, sliced

6 red peppers, halved,
    cored and deseeded

2 tbsp olive oil

2 medium tomatoes,
    finely diced

3 hard-boiled eggs

2 tbsp capers

2 tbsp sliced green olives

2 tbsp chopped parsley leaves

2 tbsp oregano leaves

salt and black pepper

Dressing

2 tbsp olive oil

zest and juice of 1 lemon

1 tsp sherry vinegar

ROAST RED PEPPER & EGG SALAD

Both eggs and red peppers are good brain food. Eggs really are a super-food, full of vitamins and minerals and also an excellent source of a nutrient called choline, which plays a role in brain health. This salad is nice as a starter or can be served over toast or bread or on little gem leaves.

Put the red onion slices in a bowl of salted water and leave to soak for 30 minutes.

Preheat the oven to 200°C/Fan 180°C/Gas 6. Toss the peppers in the oil and put them in a roasting tin. Roast for about half an hour, until the pepper skins start to blister. Remove them from the oven, put the peppers in a bowl and cover with a plate. Leave the peppers to cool and when they're cool enough to handle, remove as much of the skins as you can. Tear the flesh into thick strips.

Arrange the peppers on 4 plates. Sprinkle over the drained red onion slices and the diced tomatoes. Whisk the dressing ingredients together. Season the vegetables with salt and pepper, then pour over the dressing.

Peel the eggs and separate into whites and yolks. Finely chop the whites and crumble the yolks. Sprinkle the whites, then the yolks over the vegetables. Top with the capers, olives, parsley and oregano leaves.

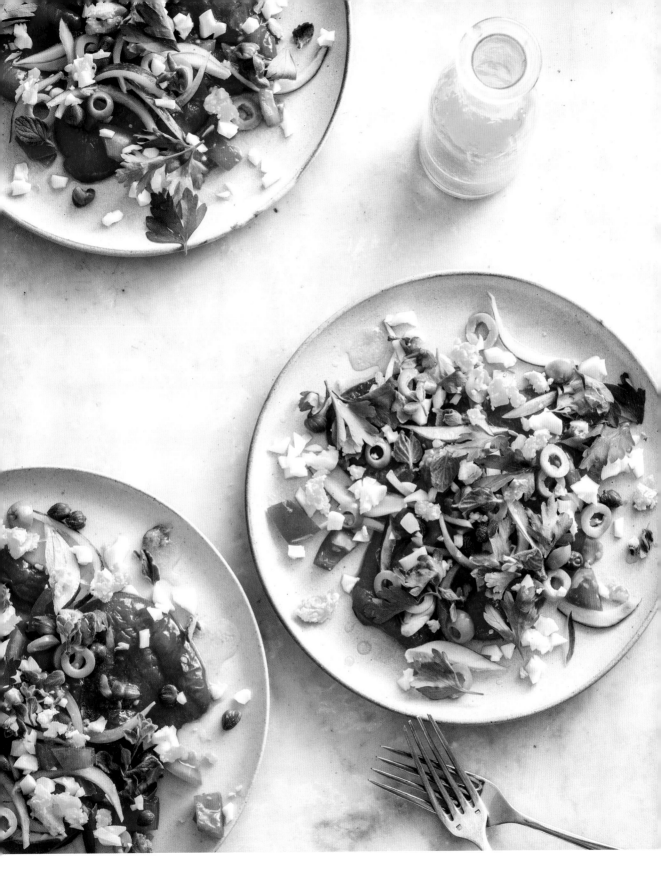

INFO PER SERVING: CALORIES 233 PROTEIN (G) 6.5 CARBS (G) 14 SUGAR (G) 13 FAT (G) 15 SATURATED FAT (G) 2.5 FIBRE (G) 7 SALT (G) 0.3

2 tbsp olive oil, plus extra
    to drizzle
1 small onion, finely chopped
2 leeks, finely sliced
1 medium floury potato, finely
    diced (no need to peel)
2 garlic cloves, finely chopped
zest and juice of 1 lemon
1 tbsp almond butter
1 litre vegetable stock
200g fresh or frozen spinach
    (no need to defrost first)
salt and black pepper

To serve
2 tbsp flaked almonds,
    lightly toasted

LEEK, SPINACH & ALMOND SOUP

Popeye ate spinach to boost his muscle power, but the research suggests it's good for your brain too, and adding lemon zest and juice helps the body absorb the iron. Both leeks and almonds are also nutrient rich.

Heat the olive oil in a large saucepan and add the onion, leeks and potato. Season with salt and pepper, stir to combine, then add a splash of water and cover the pan. Leave to cook gently for about 15 minutes until just cooked through, stirring regularly.

Add the garlic to the pan and cook for a further minute. Stir in the lemon zest, followed by the almond butter, then pour in the stock. Stir until everything is well combined, then add the spinach, pushing it down into the stock until wilted if you're using fresh. Bring to the boil, then turn the heat down and simmer for up to another 10 minutes, until everything is completely tender.

Blend the soup using a stick or jug blender. Taste for seasoning and adjust, then add lemon juice to taste – the lemon helps you absorb the iron in the spinach. Serve drizzled with a little olive oil and garnished with the flaked almonds.

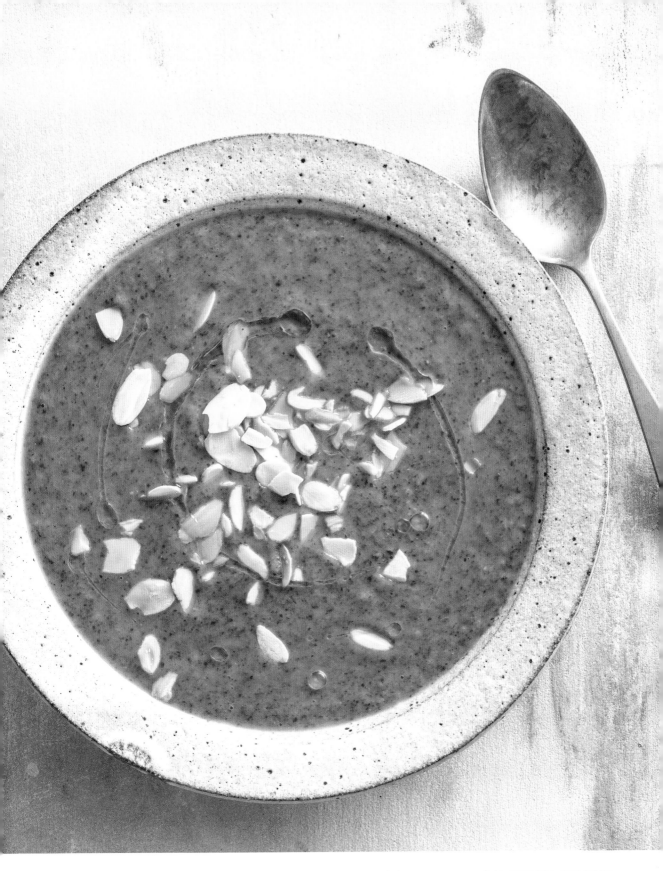

INFO PER SERVING: CALORIES 218 PROTEIN (G) 7 CARBS (G) 15 SUGAR (G) 6 FAT (G) 13 SATURATED FAT (G) 2 FIBRE (G) 6 SALT (G) 0.3

SPICED SPLIT PEA SOUP

250g split peas, soaked overnight

1 tbsp coconut or olive oil

1 onion, very finely chopped

1 sweet potato, finely chopped

15g root ginger, peeled and very finely chopped

3 garlic cloves, finely chopped

2 tbsp finely chopped coriander stems

1 tsp ground turmeric

½ tsp ground cinnamon

½ tsp cayenne or hot chilli powder

800ml vegetable stock

400ml can of coconut milk

salt and black pepper

To serve

lime juice

coriander leaves

Split pea is one of our favourite soups, but we do find the peas vary a lot in the time they take to cook, so it's a good idea to soak them before using. Turmeric may help brain function – add plenty of black pepper too, as it helps your body absorb the spice.

Drain the soaked split peas. Heat the oil in a large saucepan, add the onion and sauté until soft and translucent. Add the sweet potato, ginger and garlic and cook for another couple of minutes. Stir in the coriander stems, spices and split peas, then pour in the stock. Season with salt and plenty of black pepper.

Cover and bring to the boil, then turn the heat down and simmer for 10 minutes. Add the coconut milk and bring to the boil again, then turn down to a simmer and cook until the split peas have softened and broken down into the liquid. This might take anything from 30 minutes to an hour depending on how old the split peas are.

Check for seasoning and texture – if the soup is a little thick, you can add more liquid. Serve with a squeeze of lime juice and a sprinkle of coriander leaves.

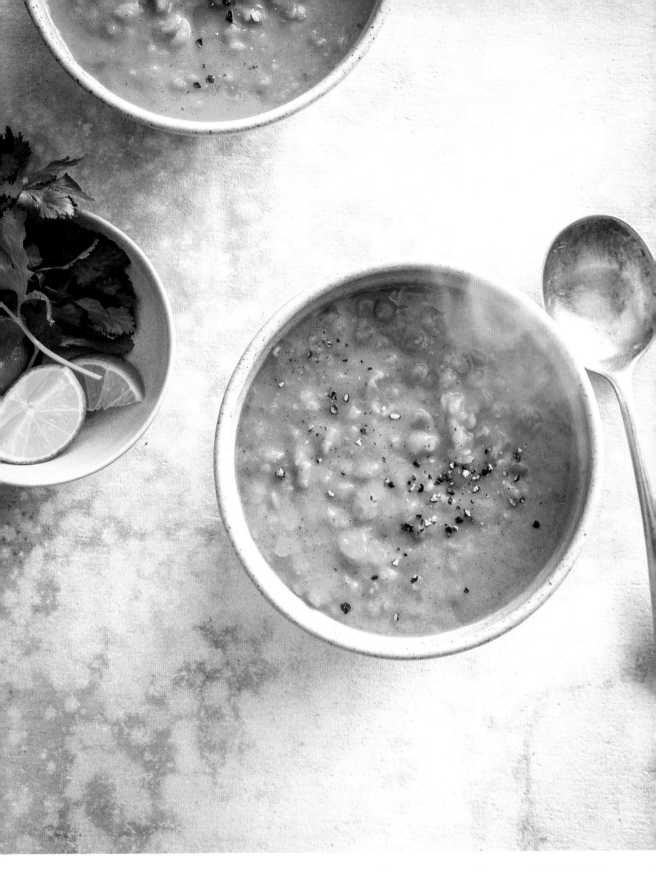

INFO PER SERVING: CALORIES 385 PROTEIN (G) 8.5 CARBS (G) 37 SUGAR (G) 11 FAT (G) 21 SATURATED FAT (G) 17.5 FIBRE (G) 6.5 SALT (G) 0.2

400g new/salad potatoes,
cut into chunks, if large

400g sprouting broccoli,
trimmed

4 spring onions, finely chopped

1 large gherkin, finely chopped
(optional)

small bunch of dill, finely
chopped

100–130g baby spinach, rocket
and/or watercress

1 tbsp olive oil

1 tsp white wine vinegar

100g cherry tomatoes, halved

salt and black pepper

Tuna dressing

1 can of tuna in oil (about 100g
drained weight)

1 tbsp capers

1 garlic clove, finely chopped

juice of 1 lemon

1 tbsp mayonnaise

1 tbsp crème fraiche or
soured cream

WARM POTATO & BROCCOLI SALAD WITH TUNA DRESSING

We were inspired by the Italian classic tuna tonnato to create what we think is an epic dressing for this salad. It makes a nice alternative to the regular potato salad.

First cook the potatoes and broccoli. Put the potatoes in a steamer and cook them over simmering water for 15 minutes, until tender. Add the sprouting broccoli for the last 5 minutes, but check after 3 minutes to see if it's tender to the point of a knife.

While the vegetables are cooking, make the tuna dressing. Put the tuna, capers, garlic and lemon juice into a small food processor or blender and blitz until smooth. Add the mayonnaise and crème fraiche or soured cream and season with plenty of salt and pepper. Blend again and the texture will loosen up to a pourable sauce.

Separate the potatoes and broccoli. Add the spring onions, the gherkin, if using, and half the dill to the warm potatoes, then drizzle over a tablespoon of the tuna dressing along with a tablespoon of water. Toss to combine.

Toss the leaves with the olive oil and vinegar and season with salt and pepper. Arrange them on a platter or in 4 shallow salad bowls. Add the potatoes, sprouting broccoli and cherry tomatoes, then drizzle over the remaining dressing. Garnish with the rest of the dill and serve while still warm.

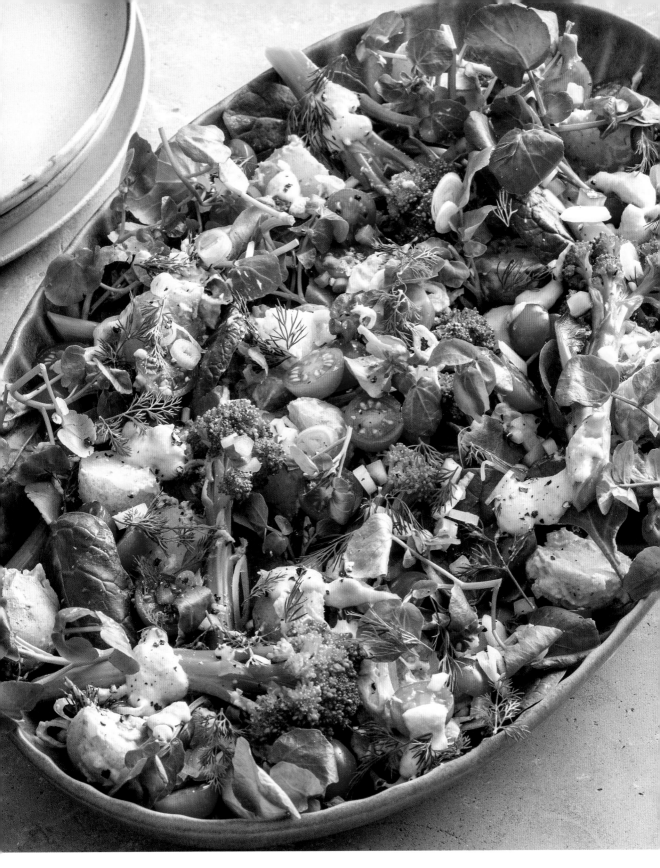

INFO PER SERVING: CALORIES 241 PROTEIN (G) 13 CARBS (G) 20 SUGAR (G) 5 FAT (G) 10 SATURATED FAT (G) 2 FIBRE (G) 7.5 SALT (G) 0.4

Serves: **4**

Prep: **10 minutes**

Cooking time: **5 minutes**

SARDINES ON TOAST

- 2 x 120g tins sardines in spring water, drained
- 150g cherry tomatoes, halved or quartered
- ½ red onion, finely chopped
- 2 tbsp capers
- leaves from a fresh oregano sprig, chopped, or ½ tsp dried oregano
- 2 tsp red wine vinegar
- juice and zest of ½ lemon
- 4 large slices of sourdough bread, toasted
- 1 garlic clove, halved (optional)
- 1 tbsp olive oil
- salt and black pepper

To serve

- rocket leaves
- olive oil
- lemon juice

Oily fish contains omega-3 which is important for brain health. Take your sardines up a notch with this quick and easy recipe – a great way to get your oily fish fix.

Put the sardines in a bowl and mash them roughly. Add the cherry tomatoes, red onion, capers and oregano, then drizzle over the red wine vinegar, lemon juice and zest. Taste for seasoning and add salt and pepper as necessary.

Take the slices of toasted sourdough and rub them with garlic, if using. Drizzle with olive oil – a tablespoon should be enough for all 4 slices. Top with the sardine mixture followed by a handful of rocket. Drizzle with a little more olive oil and a squeeze of lemon juice, then serve at once.

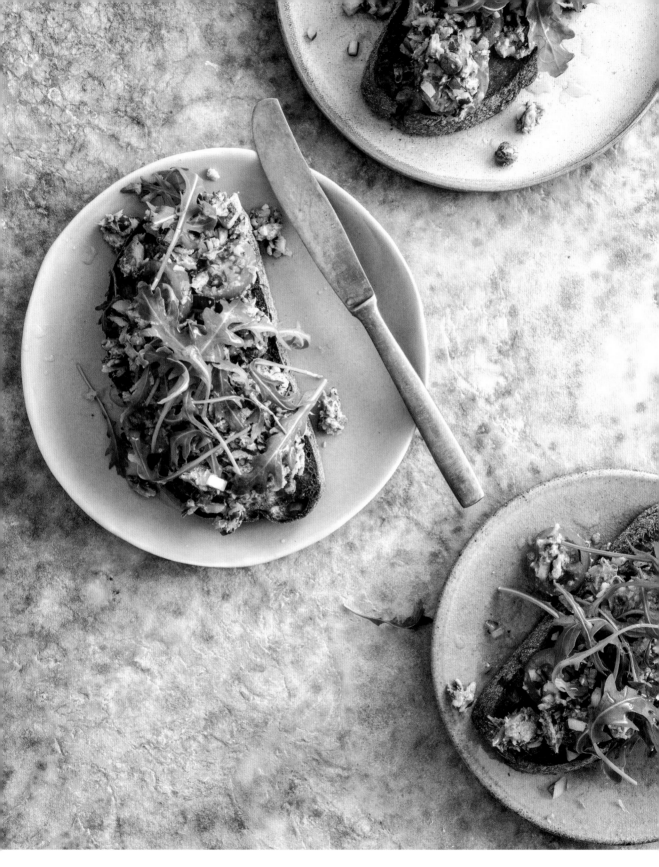

INFO PER SERVING: CALORIES 272 PROTEIN (G) 19 CARBS (G) 26 SUGAR (G) 4 FAT (G) 9.5 SATURATED FAT (G) 2 FIBRE (G) 2.5 SALT (G) 0.6

2 large boneless chicken
    breasts
zest and juice of 1 lemon
1 tbsp olive oil
1 tsp dried oregano
salt and black pepper

Sauce
1 tbsp olive oil
1 small onion, finely chopped
2 garlic cloves, finely chopped
100g walnuts, chopped
leaves from 1 thyme sprig
leaves from 2 tarragon sprigs
a few parsley sprigs
½ tsp ground allspice
2 tsp red wine vinegar
1 tsp Dijon mustard

To serve (optional)
pitta
lettuce
tomatoes

GRILLED CHICKEN WITH WALNUT SAUCE

All nuts are good brain food but walnuts are said to be the best of all, as they have the highest level of omega-3. This nutty sauce does taste quite sharp on its own but it works really well with the chicken. Nice served just with a salad and also good as a perfectly stuffed pitta with lettuce and tomato. Slicing the chicken breasts in half helps them cook quickly and stay tender.

First prepare the chicken breasts. Place one on the work surface and slice through it from one long side to the other. Cut all the way through so you have 2 pieces with the same surface area but half the thickness. Repeat with the other breast.

Season the chicken breasts with salt and pepper. Whisk the lemon zest and juice with the olive oil and add the oregano. Pour this over the chicken and then mix – preferably with your hands – to make sure the chicken is evenly coated. Leave it to marinate while you make the sauce.

To make the sauce, heat the olive oil in a small frying pan and add the onion. Cook until translucent, then turn up the heat and fry until lightly browned. Add the garlic and walnuts and cook for a further couple of minutes or until the walnuts smell toasted and aromatic. Transfer to a food processor.

Add the herbs, allspice, vinegar and mustard to the food processor and season with plenty of salt and pepper. Process in short bursts at first to break everything down, then while the motor is running, gradually add water – up to about 100ml – to make a smooth, thick, creamy sauce. Transfer to a small serving bowl.

To cook the chicken, heat a griddle pan and add the chicken. Cook for 3–4 minutes on each side until cooked through with deep char lines. Serve the chicken with the sauce and salad or pitta.

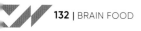

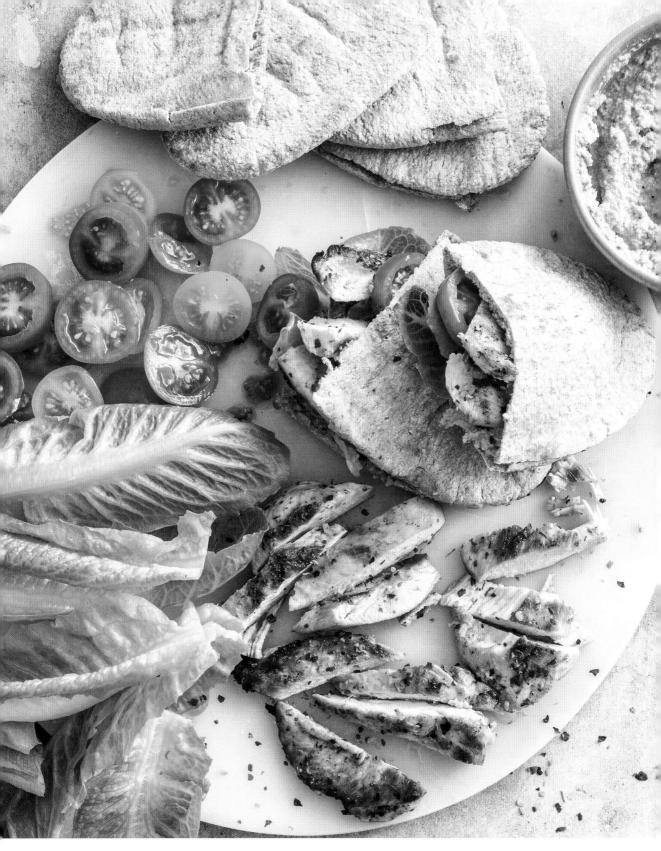

INFO PER SERVING (CHICKEN AND SAUCE):   CALORIES 344   PROTEIN (G) 29   CARBS (G) 3   SUGAR (G) 2   FAT (G) 24

SATURATED FAT (G) 3   FIBRE (G) 2   SALT (G) 0.3

1 tbsp olive oil

1 red onion, sliced

400g chicken livers

200g cooked lentils
(80g uncooked weight)

1 orange, peeled and divided
into segments

200g cavolo nero, shredded

salt and black pepper

Sauce

1 tbsp red wine vinegar

2 red chillies, finely chopped

25g root ginger, finely chopped
or grated

2 garlic cloves, finely chopped

zest of ½ an orange

juice of 2 oranges

100ml chicken stock

To serve

a few parsley sprigs

a few mint sprigs

CHICKEN LIVERS WITH LEAFY GREENS

A light but very nourishing one-pot meal, this would also work well with green beans or sprouting broccoli. Chicken livers are cheap, low in calories and high in protein, as well as being a good source of brain-boosting essential fatty acids and vitamins and minerals. They're well worth including in your diet and tasty too.

First whisk the sauce ingredients together in a jug and season with salt and pepper.

Heat the oil in a large sauté pan with a lid. Add the red onion and cook over a low to medium heat until softened and starting to colour. Turn up the heat and push the onion to one side of the pan. Add the chicken livers and sear them briefly on all sides, then mix them with the onion and season with salt and pepper.

Sprinkle over the lentils, then pour the sauce into the pan. Add the orange segments, then place the cavolo nero on top. Bring to the boil, then cover the pan and leave to simmer for about 10 minutes until the chicken livers are cooked through and the cavolo nero is tender.

Serve in shallow bowls and sprinkle with the parsley and mint.

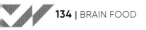

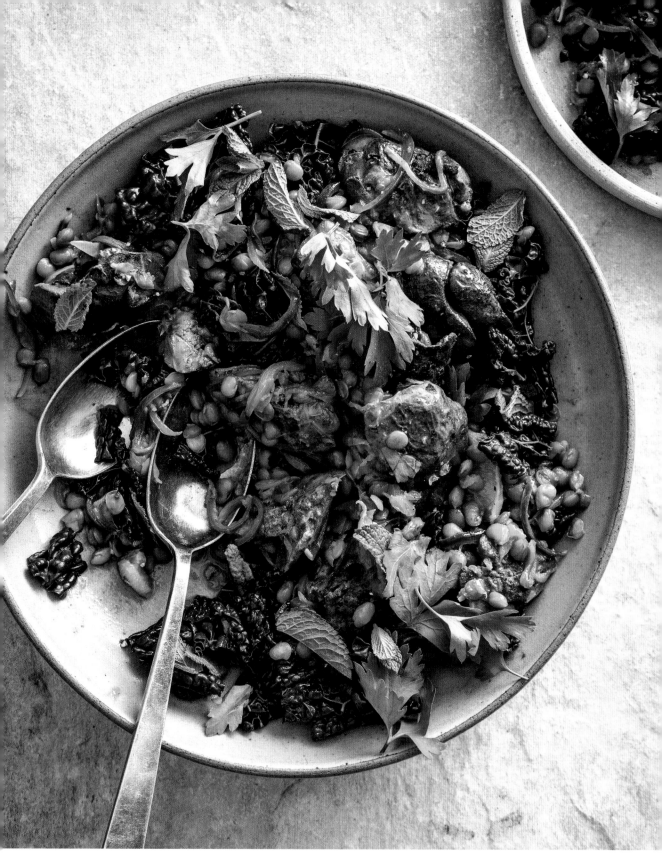

INFO PER SERVING: CALORIES 235 PROTEIN (G) 25 CARBS (G) 16 SUGAR (G) 7 FAT (G) 6.5 SATURATED FAT (G) 1.5 FIBRE (G) 6 SALT (G) 0.3

3 thin slices of root ginger

3 thin slices of fresh turmeric
   root

a few black peppercorns

2cm piece of cinnamon bark

1 tsp honey

lemon or lime slices

GINGER & TURMERIC TEA

Spicy and refreshing, this makes a healthy alternative to your regular cuppa. Ginger is a great anti-inflammatory, while turmeric is said to boost brain power. Be sure to include the black pepper as it helps the absorption of turmeric. We like to take a flask of this for elevenses when we're out on our bikes filming.

Put the ginger, turmeric, peppercorns and cinnamon in a mug (or in a mug infuser if you want to remove the spices before drinking). Muddle gently with a pestle, making sure the peppercorns are lightly crushed.

Pour over freshly boiled hot water and stir in honey to taste. Add slices of lemon or lime and leave to steep for at least 5 minutes before drinking. Then, if you like, top up with more freshly boiled hot water and enjoy again

 Tip: To make this really quick and easy, thinly slice some turmeric and ginger and store them in the freezer. Then you can make yourself a cuppa whenever you fancy with very little effort.

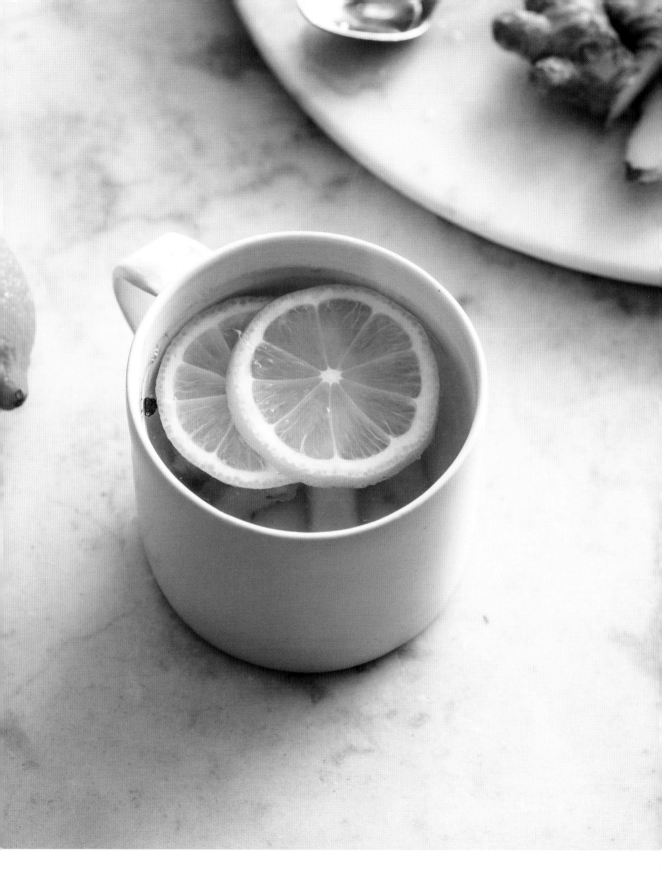

INFO PER SERVING: CALORIES 23 PROTEIN (G) 0 CARBS (G) 6 SUGAR (G) 6 FAT (G) 0 SATURATED FAT (G) 0 FIBRE (G) 0 SALT (G) 0

75ml olive oil, plus extra
    for greasing
125ml live yoghurt
75g well-flavoured honey
1 tsp vanilla extract
3 eggs
75g golden caster sugar
125g ground almonds
100g plain flour
½ tsp ground cinnamon
2 tsp baking powder
pinch of salt
150g blueberries

BLUEBERRY MINI LOAF CAKES

This is a celebration of blueberries – the healthiest of all berries. They're low in calories but high in antioxidants and rich in vitamins K and C. We like making these as mini loaf cakes – that way we're not tempted to cut a big slice – but you could also bake them in cupcake tins. Great for popping into your lunch box.

Preheat the oven to 200°C/Fan 180°C/Gas 6. Lightly grease a 12-hole mini loaf tin with a little oil.

Put the olive oil, yoghurt, honey, vanilla extract and eggs into a large bowl and beat together until smooth.

Put the sugar, ground almonds, flour, cinnamon and baking powder into a separate bowl with a generous pinch of salt. Mix thoroughly, then add to the wet ingredients. Stir to combine – you will end up with quite a runny batter.

Spoon the cake batter into the 12 holes, then divide the blueberries evenly between them, leaving them sitting on top.

Bake for about 20 minutes until the cakes are well risen around the blueberries and have turned a rich golden brown. Leave to cool in the tin, then turn out and store in an airtight container.

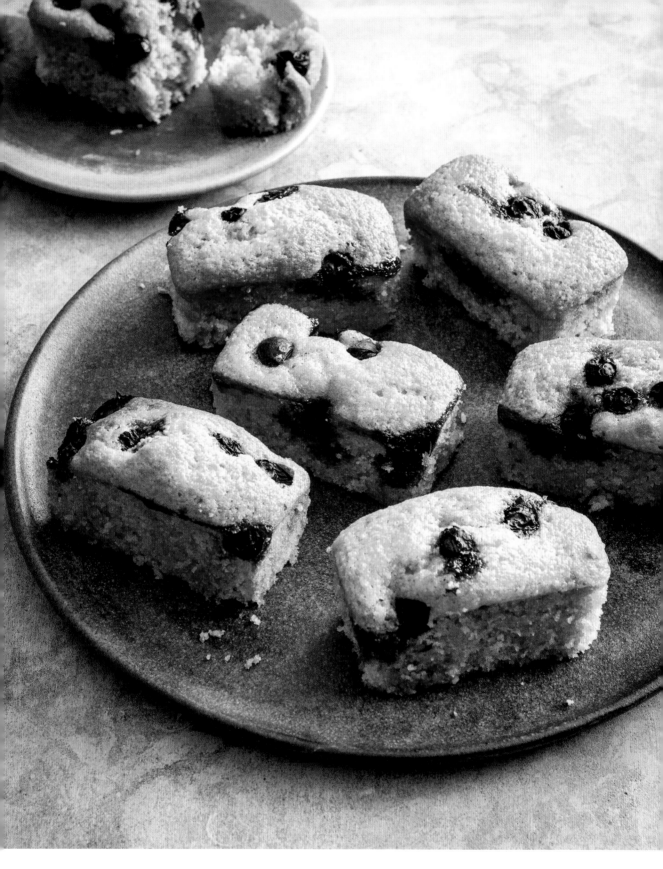

INFO PER CAKE: CALORIES 216   PROTEIN (G) 6   CARBS (G) 20   SUGAR (G) 13   FAT (G) 12   SATURATED FAT (G) 2   FIBRE (G) 0.5   SALT (G) 0.4

LOOK AFTER YOUR HEART

A good diet is all-important for your heart health and that means cutting right down on processed foods and upping your intake of fruit, vegetables, whole grains and pulses. We know that we should limit our intake of high-fat dairy products to keep our cholesterol in check, but we do need good fats for a healthy heart – foods such as oily fish, nuts and olive oil. Beans and pulses and foods rich in soluble fibre will all help reduce cholesterol levels. We've also been experimenting with tofu, which is a really heart-friendly ingredient and have come up with a couple of dishes we think you're going to love. And we've even made a chocolate and almond cake that contains no butter but is still a delicious treat.

200g porridge oats

1 tbsp chia seeds

1 tbsp sesame seeds

50g whole, unskinned almonds,
   roughly chopped

100g mixed dried fruit
   (raisins, sultanas,
   chopped prunes, apricots)

½ tsp ground cinnamon

pinch of salt

To serve

200ml whole milk (dairy
   or plant-based)

100ml yoghurt or kefir (dairy
   or plant-based)

200g fresh berries left whole
   or 4 orchard fruits, cored
   or pitted and diced

honey or maple syrup

OVERNIGHT OATS WITH FRUIT & NUTS

Oats are great for reducing your cholesterol levels and we've heard that steel-cut oats are even better for you than rolled oats, so maybe give them a try? Add any seeds you like to this mixture, but be careful at first if you're not used to them. Your digestive system might need time to adapt. If you use flax seeds, always grind them first.

The night before you want to eat your oats, put them in a container with the seeds, almonds, dried fruit and cinnamon. Add a pinch of salt and mix thoroughly, then pour over 500ml of water. Cover and leave in the fridge overnight.

When you are ready to eat, stir in the milk. Add yoghurt or kefir and some fruit to each bowl, then top with a drizzle of honey or maple syrup for a touch of extra sweetness.

Tip: This recipe is a year-round treat. In summer, fresh fruit is great with this, but in winter, if you have berries in the freezer, try adding some to the mixture before refrigerating and they will defrost overnight. You might also like to warm the oats gently, then add hot milk just before serving.

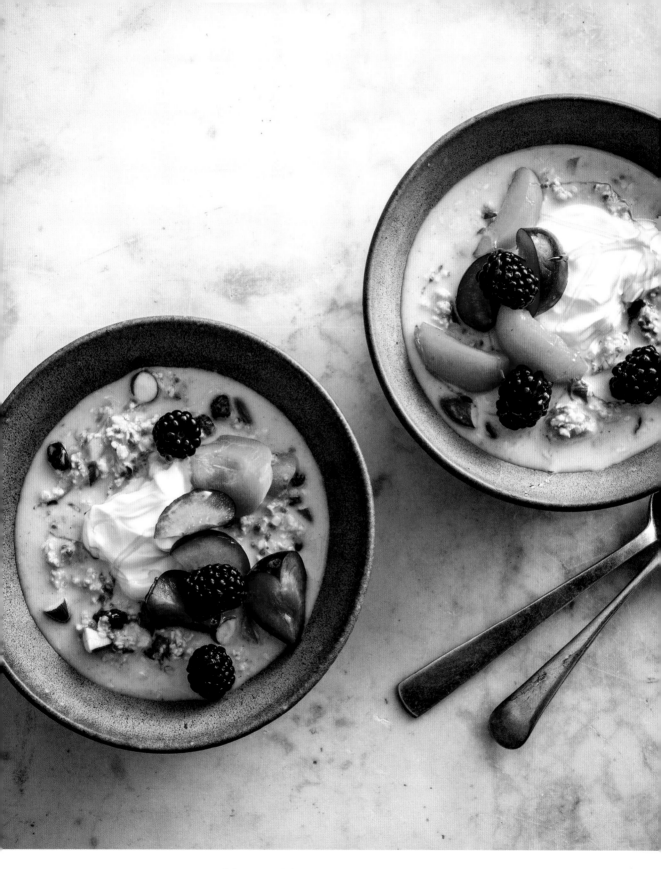

INFO PER SERVING: CALORIES 445 PROTEIN (G) 12 CARBS (G) 61 SUGAR (G) 25 FAT (G) 15 SATURATED FAT (G) 2 FIBRE (G) 7 SALT (G) TRACE

KOREAN RICE BOWL

2 tsp olive or vegetable oil

1 red pepper, cut into strips

130g baby corn, halved
    lengthways

100g mange tout, shredded

150g brown rice, cooked
    according to the packet
    instructions

150g soybeans, blanched

100g radishes, sliced

1 tbsp soy sauce

chopped fresh coriander

bunch of spring onions,
    halved and shredded

4 eggs, fried or poached
    (optional)

1 tsp sesame seeds

Sauce

1 tsp gochugaru or other
    chilli flakes

2 tbsp soy sauce

1 tbsp rice vinegar

1 tsp honey

1 tsp sesame oil

2 garlic cloves, finely chopped

10g root ginger, grated

salt and black pepper

To serve

250g kimchi (shop-bought
    or see p.182)

Korean food really packs a punch. We both love it and dishes like this are both great to eat and super healthy. There's a tasty selection of vegetables here and the optional egg adds extra protein and deliciousness.

First make the sauce. Whisk everything together and taste, then add more chilli flakes to taste and season with salt and pepper as necessary.

Heat the oil in a frying pan or wok. When it's hot, add the pepper, baby corn and mange tout and stir-fry until everything is softened but still has a little bite. Remove the pan from the heat.

Divide the cooked vegetables, rice, soybeans and radishes between 4 bowls and drizzle over a little soy sauce.

Mix the coriander and spring onions together and dress with half the sauce, then toss thoroughly. Drizzle the remaining sauce over the contents of the bowls, then add the coriander and spring onions. Top with the fried or poached eggs, if using, and a sprinkling of sesame seeds. Serve with plenty of kimchi on the side.

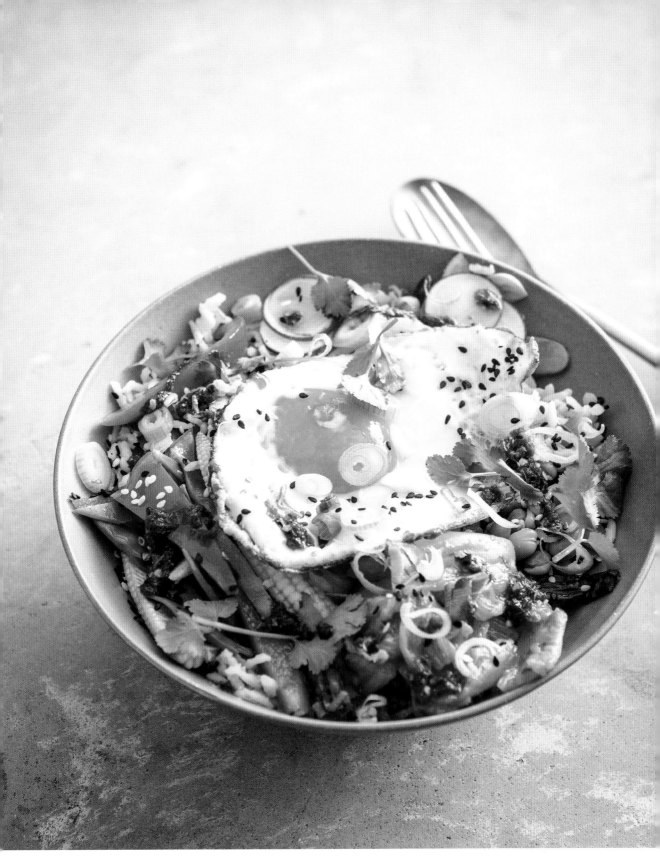

INFO PER SERVING: CALORIES 365 PROTEIN (G) 19 CARBS (G) 40 SUGAR (G) 7 FAT (G) 12.5 SATURATED FAT (G) 2.5 FIBRE (G) 7 SALT (G) 3.3

Serves: **4–6**　　　Prep: **see below**　　　Cooking time: **see below**

Prep: **5 minutes**

400g can of black beans,
　　drained
2 tsp tahini
1 garlic clove, grated
zest and juice of 1 lime
½ tsp dried oregano
½ tsp ground cumin
½ tsp ground cinnamon
1 tsp chilli paste or sauce
2 tbsp olive oil
salt and black pepper

To garnish
1 tbsp olive oil
½ tsp chilli paste or sauce
finely chopped coriander
　　leaves

TRIO OF HUMMUS

All these dips are good heart-friendly snack options to have in the fridge when hunger pangs strike or to take to work for lunch. Serve with pitta bread, tortilla chips or sticks of raw veg.

BLACK BEAN HUMMUS

Put the black beans in a food processor with the tahini, garlic, lime zest and juice, oregano, spices and chilli paste or sauce. Season with salt and pepper. Process until well combined but not completely smooth – you want to keep some texture and the mixture should be slightly flecked with black from the beans. Drizzle in the olive oil while the motor is still running, then transfer to a bowl.

For the garnish, whisk the olive oil with the chilli paste or sauce. Sprinkle the coriander over the top of the hummus, then drizzle over the oil.

Prep: **10 minutes**

Cooking time: **25 minutes**

2 tbsp olive oil
200g carrots, sliced finely
　　on the diagonal
100g red lentils, well rinsed
½ tsp cinnamon
½ tsp turmeric
½ tsp ground coriander
25g walnuts, finely chopped
1 garlic clove, grated
2 tsp tahini
zest and juice of ½ lemon
salt and black pepper

CARROT, RED LENTIL & WALNUT HUMMUS

Put the olive oil in a sauté pan with a lid. Heat until hot, then add the carrots. Sauté over a high heat until lightly browned, then add a splash of water, cover the pan and leave the carrots to braise until tender. Drain and leave to cool.

At the same time, put the red lentils in a saucepan and cover with 250ml of water. Season with plenty of salt and bring to the boil, then cover the pan and turn down the heat to a simmer. Cook until all the water has been absorbed, stirring every so often to make sure the lentils aren't catching. When the lentils have collapsed into a thick purée, remove the lid and leave over a very low heat for a few more minutes until they have a slightly drier consistency. Remove from the heat and leave to cool.

Put the spices and walnuts in a food processor and pulse until the nuts are quite finely ground. Add the garlic, cooked carrots, tahini, lemon zest and juice and continue to process until the carrots have broken down. Add the red lentils and process again to combine. Taste and add plenty of salt and pepper.

AVOCADO HUMMUS

Prep: **5 minutes**

400g can of chickpeas, drained

1 ripe avocado, peeled and diced

zest and juice of 1 lime

1 tsp tahini

1 garlic clove, grated

½ tsp ground cumin

2 tbsp finely chopped coriander
    stems, keep leaves for garnish

olive oil

pinch of chilli flakes

salt and black pepper

Put the chickpeas in a food processor and pulse until they start to break up. Toss the avocado in the lime zest and juice, then add this to the food processor along with the tahini, garlic, cumin and coriander stems. Season with plenty of salt and pepper.

Process to a fairly smooth purée, then drizzle in a tablespoon of olive oil while the motor is running until it's all combined. Taste for seasoning and add more salt, pepper or lime juice as necessary. Transfer to a bowl. Sprinkle over the coriander leaves and chilli flakes and drizzle over more olive oil.

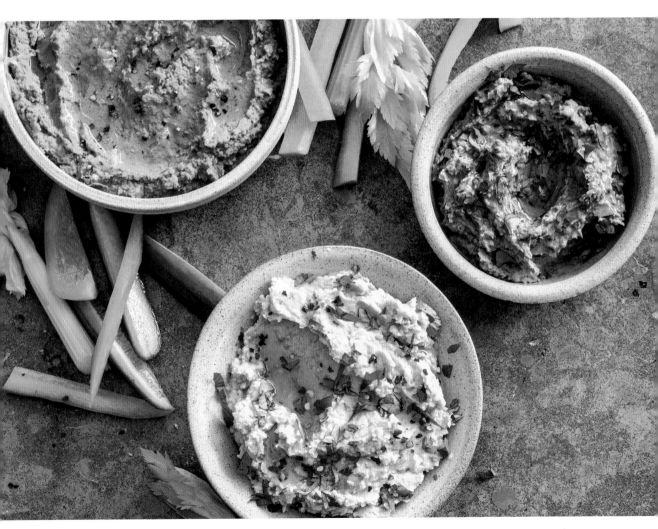

INFO PER 50G SERVING (BLACK BEAN/CARROT/AVOCADO):   CALORIES 108/158/91   PROTEIN (G) 3.5/6/3   CARBS (G) 5/12/4
SUGAR (G) 0/2/0   FAT (G) 7/9/7   SATURATED FAT (G) 1/1.5/1.25   FIBRE (G) 3.5/2.5/3   SALT (G) TRACE

CRISPY TOFU STIR-FRY

People can be funny about tofu but we love it and we've had some fantastic tofu dishes in Japan. It's high in protein but relatively low in calories and it may help reduce your cholesterol. And we think the crispy coating in this recipe really brings the tofu to life. A tasty dish and high in fibre too.

First make the sauce by whisking together all the ingredients until well combined. Season with salt and pepper.

Next prepare the tofu. Pat it dry with kitchen paper. Whisk the cornflour with the chilli powder, turmeric and five-spice powder and season with plenty of salt and black pepper. Toss the tofu in the cornflour mixture.

Bring a pan of salted water to the boil, add the green beans and cook for a couple of minutes, then drain and refresh under cold water. Set aside.

Heat 2 teaspoons of vegetable oil in a wok or large frying pan. When the air above the oil is shimmering, add the chunks of tofu and fry them on all sides until crisp and golden brown. Remove from the wok and drain on kitchen paper.

Give the wok a quick wipe and add a tablespoon of vegetable oil. When it's hot, add all the vegetables, including the green beans, and stir-fry until just al dente. Add the garlic and cook for another minute or so. Pour over the sauce and simmer until piping hot. Add the tofu and toss everything together.

Drizzle with the sesame oil. Divide between bowls (over brown rice if you like) and sprinkle with sesame seeds. Garnish with coriander and spring onions before serving.

Sauce

2 tbsp soy sauce

1 tbsp mirin

1 tbsp rice vinegar

15g root ginger, grated

1 tsp honey

salt and black pepper

Stir-fry

1 block extra-firm tofu (about 300g), cut into chunks

2 tsp cornflour

½ tsp chilli powder

½ tsp ground turmeric

½ tsp Chinese five-spice powder

200g green beans, trimmed and halved

vegetable oil

1 carrot, cut into matchsticks

100g asparagus tips

200g sprouting broccoli, trimmed and blanched

2 garlic cloves, finely chopped

To serve

1 tsp sesame oil

1 tsp sesame seeds

a few coriander sprigs

2 spring onions, shredded

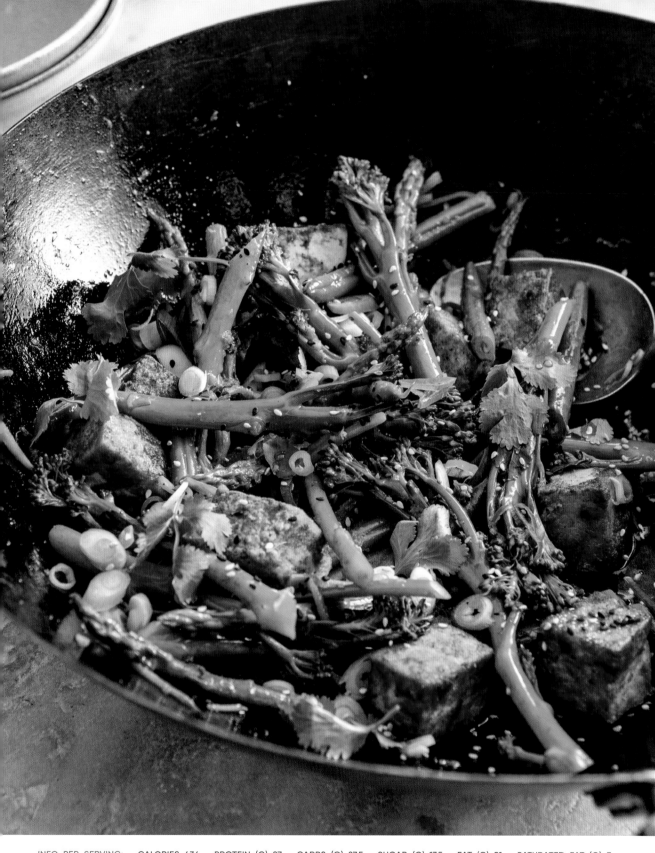

INFO PER SERVING: CALORIES 434   PROTEIN (G) 27   CARBS (G) 27.5   SUGAR (G) 17.5   FAT (G) 21   SATURATED FAT (G) 3

FIBRE (G) 14.5 SALT (G) 2.3

1 tbsp chia seeds

olive oil

1 small onion, finely chopped

2 garlic cloves, finely chopped

1 pack of extra-firm tofu (about 280g), coarsely grated

2 tbsp wholemeal flour

3 tbsp oatmeal or porridge oats

1 tsp curry powder

2 tbsp coriander stems, finely chopped

1 tbsp soy sauce

1 tbsp cornflour

salt and black pepper

To serve

100g thick yoghurt or kefir

1 tsp mint

4 burger buns

4 lettuce leaves

1 tomato, sliced

4 slices of red onion

4 slices of cucumber

TOFU BURGERS

We always like to have a burger in our books and hey presto – we bring you our Big Tof! Have a change from your regular burger and enjoy this with all the trimmings and everyone will be happy. One tip – do be sure to include the chia seeds in the mix, as they help to bind everything together.

Put the chia seeds in a small bowl and add 3 tablespoons of water. Leave until the liquid has been absorbed.

Heat a tablespoon of olive oil in a frying pan and add the onion. Sauté over a medium heat until it's translucent and starting to brown, then add the garlic and cook for a further minute. Transfer to a food processor.

Add the tofu, flour, oatmeal, curry powder and coriander stems to the food processor and season with salt and pepper. Process to bring everything together, then tip the mixture into a bowl. Mix the soy sauce with the swollen chia seeds and add this to the bowl. Stir well, then form the mixture into 4 patties. Dust the patties with cornflour, patting off any excess.

Heat a little more oil in a frying pan and add the patties. Fry them for a few minutes on each side, putting a lid on the pan towards the end of the cooking time just to help the burgers heat through.

To serve, mix the yoghurt with the mint. Serve the patties in buns with the salad and some of the yoghurt.

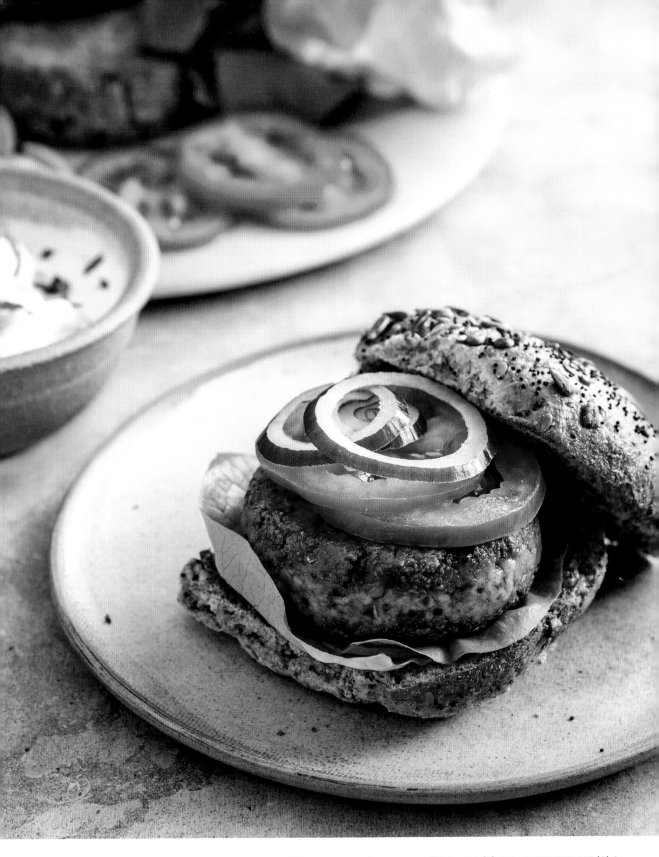

INFO PER SERVING (WITH BUN):   CALORIES 404   PROTEIN (G) 13   CARBS (G) 55   SUGAR (G) 8   FAT (G) 12.5   SATURATED FAT (G) 2

FIBRE (G) 8.5   SALT (G) 1.4

Fishcakes

3 x 125g tins of mackerel (about 82g drained weight)

1 small onion, very finely chopped

½ tsp mixed dried herbs

1 tbsp mustard

½ tsp chilli flakes

zest of 1 lemon

1 tsp cider vinegar

1 egg

40g oats, ground to a coarse flour

1 tbsp olive oil, for frying

lemon wedges, to serve

To coat

25g oats

Remoulade

1 small celeriac, peeled and cut into matchsticks

1 crisp apple, cored and coarsely grated

juice of 1 lemon

1 tsp cider or white wine vinegar

1 small onion, very finely chopped

50g crème fraiche

1 tbsp Dijon mustard

a few parsley sprigs, finely chopped

leaves from 2 tarragon sprigs, finely chopped

pinch of sugar (optional)

salt and black pepper

MACKEREL FISHCAKES WITH CELERIAC REMOULADE

Tinned fish is cheap and good for you so we've come up with a new fishcake recipe using mackerel. It works brilliantly and both oily fish and oats are very heart-healthy ingredients. This tangy celeriac salad is the perfect partner to cut through the richness of the fish. You do need to allow time for a bit of chilling and soaking for this dish, but you can get all that done in advance, then cook the fishcakes at the last minute.

Drain the mackerel and put it in a bowl. Mash or flake the fish, then add all of the remaining ingredients, except the oil, and mix thoroughly. The best way to do this is to knead the mixture with your hands. It will feel quite wet to start with, but the oats will quickly absorb liquid and help firm it up. Shape the mixture into 8 patties.

Put the 25g of oats in a small processor or grinder and give them a quick whizz to break them up a little. Tip the oats into a shallow bowl, then dip the fishcakes into them. Pat off the excess, then chill the fishcakes for half an hour.

To make the remoulade, toss the celeriac and apple in a teaspoon of salt and half the lemon juice, then leave to drain in a colander for half an hour. Put the remaining lemon juice and vinegar into a bowl with the onion, crème fraiche, mustard and herbs. Whisk everything together and taste. Season with salt, pepper and a pinch of sugar, if using. Stir in the celeriac and apple, making sure they are completely coated with the dressing.

When you are ready to cook the fishcakes, heat the oil in a large frying pan. Fry the fishcakes over a medium heat until lightly browned and heated through. Serve with the celeriac remoulade.

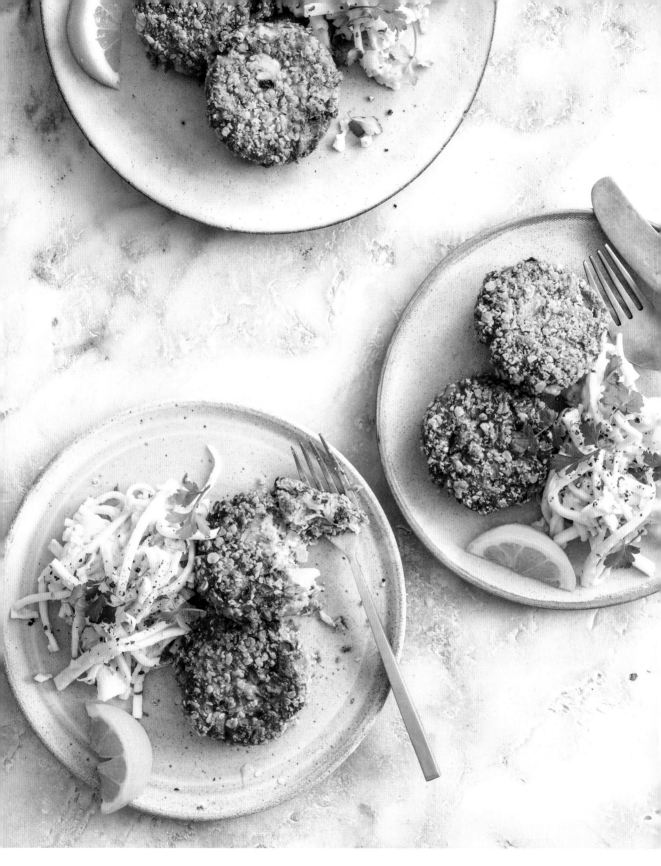

INFO PER SERVING: CALORIES 386 PROTEIN (G) 19 CARBS (G) 20 SUGAR (G) 9 FAT (G) 24 SATURATED FAT (G) 6.5 FIBRE (G) 8 SALT (G) 1.5

Marinade

2 tbsp miso paste

2 tbsp soy sauce

1 tbsp mirin or rice wine

1 tsp rice vinegar

1 tsp honey

2 garlic cloves, grated

10g root ginger, grated

salt and black pepper

Tray bake

4 salmon fillets (skin on)

1 large red pepper, sliced

1 large courgette, sliced

150g baby corn

2 tsp olive oil

1 large head of broccoli, cut into small florets

1 small bunch of asparagus, trimmed

1 bunch of spring onions, trimmed and halved

To garnish

1 tsp white or black sesame seeds

coriander leaves

MISO SALMON TRAY BAKE

We're using miso more and more to bring a rich savoury flavour to food – and it's good for you. It goes particularly well with salmon in this veggie-packed, protein-rich tray bake with an Asian twist.

Preheat the oven to 200°C/Fan 180°C/Gas 6.

Put all the marinade ingredients in a bowl and season with salt and black pepper. Brush the salmon fillets liberally with marinade and set them aside for half an hour. Reserve the rest of the marinade.

Put the pepper, courgette and baby corn in a large roasting tin and pour over the olive oil. Mix thoroughly and season with salt, then roast for 10 minutes.

Add 100ml of water to the remaining marinade in the bowl and toss the broccoli in it. Add the broccoli to the roasting tin and roast for another 10 minutes.

Place the salmon fillets on top of the roast vegetables. Toss the asparagus and spring onions in the bowl of marinade, then shake off any excess and add them to the tin. Pour any remaining marinade over all the vegetables and roast for a further 10 minutes.

Remove from the oven and garnish with sesame seeds and coriander. Serve with rice or noodles, if you like.

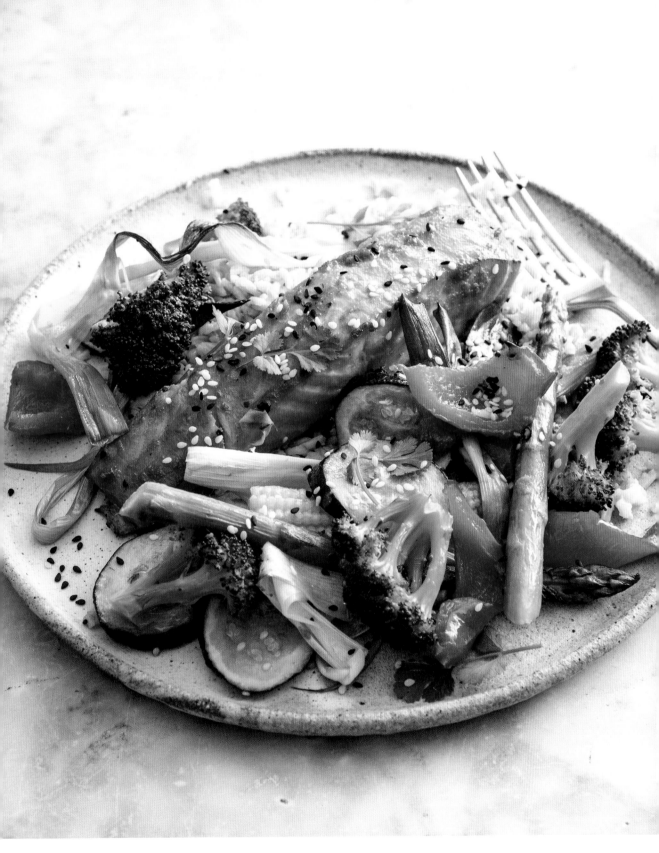

INFO PER SERVING: CALORIES 393 PROTEIN (G) 32 CARBS (G) 14 SUGAR (G) 11 FAT (G) 22 SATURATED FAT (G) 4 FIBRE (G) 6.5 SALT (G) 1.4

oil, for greasing

100g ground almonds

50g cocoa powder

½ tsp bicarbonate of soda

pinch of salt

75g runny honey

4 eggs

75g light brown soft sugar

zest of 1 orange (optional)

1 tsp vanilla extract

75g dark chocolate, finely
    chopped or coarsely grated

25g flaked almonds (optional)

CHOCOLATE & ALMOND CAKE

We do like a bit of cake every now and then and this one is low in saturated fat, so not too bad in heart terms for the occasional treat. The cake is lovely served warm with some crème fraiche, but it's good cold too and it does become more moist in texture after a day or two.

Preheat the oven to 160°C/Fan 140°C/Gas 3. Grease a 20cm round cake tin with oil and line it with baking parchment.

Put the ground almonds, cocoa powder and bicarbonate of soda in a bowl with a pinch of salt and whisk them together.

Put the honey in a separate bowl and whisk to loosen it. Beat in the eggs, followed by the sugar and the orange zest, if using, and mix thoroughly until well combined. Add the vanilla extract.

Fold the dry ingredients into the wet to make a rich dark brown batter – it will be quite runny – then stir in the chocolate. Scrape the batter into the prepared tin.

Bake the cake for about 30 minutes until springy to the touch and slightly shrunk in from the sides. Remove from the oven, turn it out on to a plate and sprinkle with the flaked almonds. This is good served warm with crème fraiche, but it will keep for up to a week in an airtight tin.

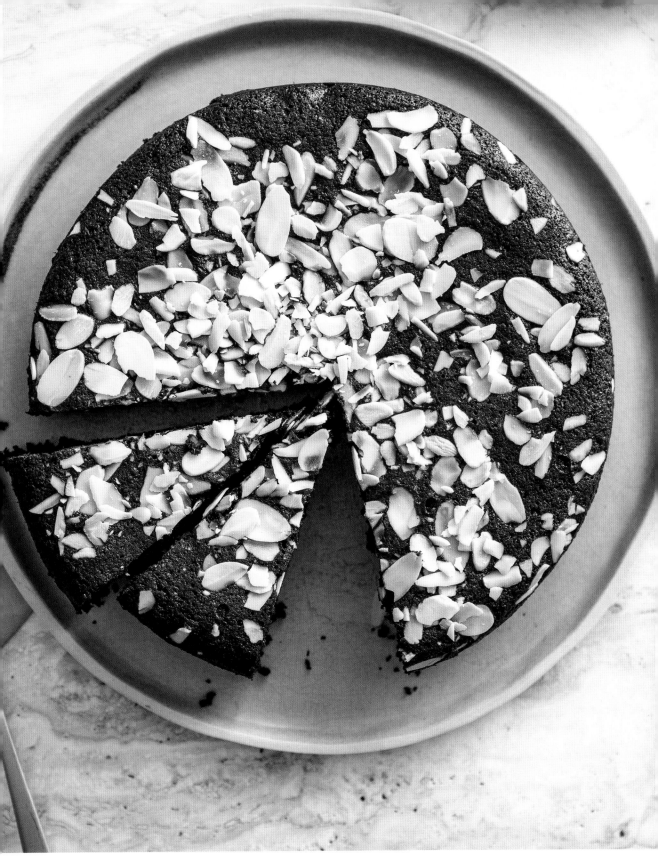

INFO PER SLICE: CALORIES 170   PROTEIN (G) 6   CARBS (G) 15   SUGAR (G) 14.5   FAT (G) 9   SATURATED FAT (G) 2.5   FIBRE (G) 1   SALT (G) 0.3

SLEEP SUPPERS

Eating the right things can even help improve your night's rest and it turns out that granny's hot milky drinks really are a good idea for soothing you at the end of the day. Milk contains an amino acid called tryptophan and this aids in the production of hormones such as serotonin and melatonin which regulate sleep patterns. Other foods rich in this amino acid include turkey, cherries, bananas, eggs, nuts and seeds. Carbs help too, so rice or pasta suppers are a good option – have you ever found yourself nodding off after a pasta lunch? And if you want a peaceful night, avoid tea and coffee and other caffeinated drinks late in the day.

WELSH RAREBIT

1 tbsp olive oil

1 leek, finely chopped

100g squash, peeled
and finely diced

1 garlic clove, very finely
chopped

½ tsp dried sage

50ml white wine, cider
or apple juice

1 eating apple, peeled
and grated

1 small onion or shallot,
very finely chopped

200g hard, strong-flavoured
cheese, such as mature
Cheddar, grated

1 egg, beaten

dash of Worcestershire sauce

4 large slices of sourdough
bread

Dijon mustard (optional)

salt and black pepper

Our mams used to say that eating cheese late in the day could lead to nightmares but we've never had a problem and we both find a bit of cheese on toast a really comforting supper. In this recipe we've cut down on the cheese for easier digestion close to bedtime, and the three alliums – leek, onion and garlic – give the dish a health boost. Delicious.

Heat the olive oil in a lidded sauté pan, add the leek and squash and stir until the contents of the pan look glossy. Add the garlic and sage, then pour in the wine, cider or apple juice and 50ml of water. Cover the pan and leave the vegetables to braise gently until tender. Make sure the squash has broken down – mash it with the back of a spoon, if necessary. Season with salt and pepper.

Stir in the apple and onion, then remove the pan from the heat and add the cheese, beaten egg and a dash of Worcestershire sauce. Mix thoroughly

Preheat the grill. Lightly toast the bread and spread it with mustard if you want a bit of heat to your rarebit. Divide the cheese mixture between the slices of bread and grill until brown and bubbling. Serve immediately.

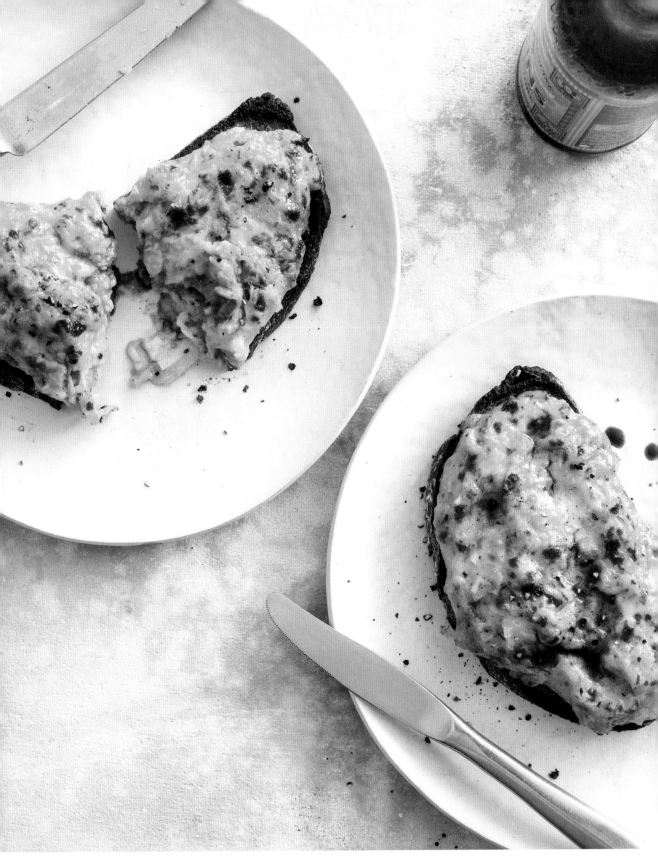

Batter

100g buckwheat flour

pinch of salt

1 egg

300ml milk

oil or butter, for frying

Filling

1 tbsp olive oil

1 tbsp (15g) butter

500g onions, sliced

1 tsp fresh thyme leaves
   or ½ tsp dried oregano

pinch of sugar (optional)

100g Gruyère, Comté
   or similar, grated

salt and black pepper

To serve

chilli flakes

thyme leaves

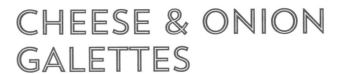

CHEESE & ONION GALETTES

Galettes or buckwheat pancakes can be sweet, but we love this savoury filling of cheese and onions which are caramelised until meltingly soft and gorgeous. You'll see we're suggesting a different method for the onions from usual – it's quicker and just as good.

First make the batter. Put the flour in a bowl with a pinch of salt and make a well. Break in the egg and work it into the flour. Add the milk, gradually at first until you have a thick batter, then whisk steadily until it is all incorporated. Set the batter aside to rest while you make the filling.

For the onions, heat the olive oil and butter in a large frying pan. Add the onions and thyme and season with salt and pepper. Stir until the onions are coated with the oil and butter, then leave to cook over a medium-high heat until they start to brown underneath and the base of the pan has a golden-brown coating. Add a couple of tablespoons of water and stir to deglaze. Repeat this several times until the onions have softened and are a deep caramelised brown – this should take 15–20 minutes.

Taste and add a pinch of sugar if you think it is needed and remove the pan from the heat. Stir the cheese into onions just to start the melting process and set aside.

Heat a large crêpe pan or frying pan and rub a little oil or butter over the base. Pour a quarter of the batter into the pan and swirl it around so the base is completely covered. Leave until the pancake has set and the underside is dappled brown, then carefully flip and cook the top side.

To assemble, put a quarter of the onion and cheese mixture in the centre of the pancake. Fold in the edges just enough to form a square, leaving most of the filling uncovered. Heat through until the cheese has melted. Garnish with a few chilli flakes and more thyme.

Repeat with the remaining batter and filling to make 4 galettes and serve at once.

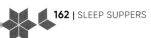

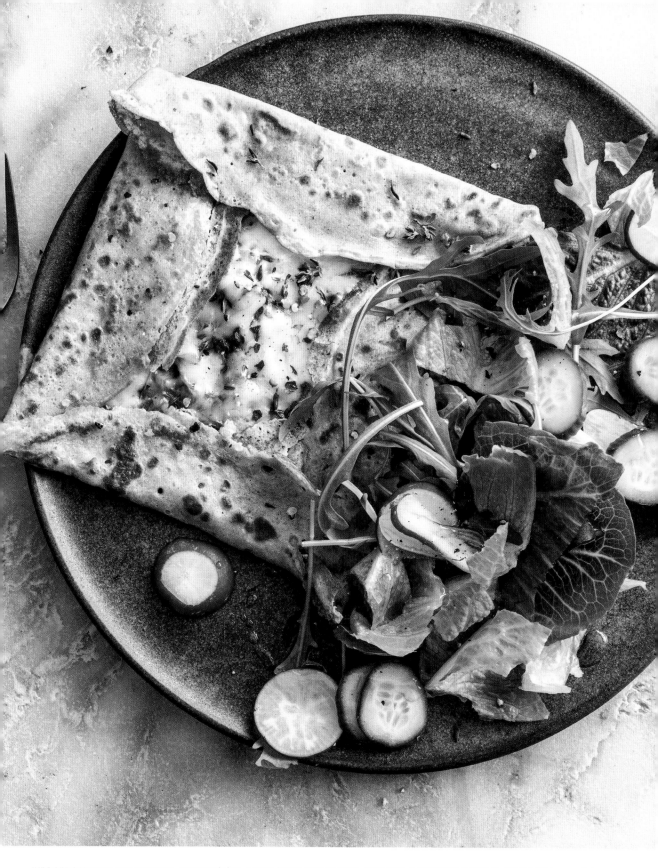

INFO PER SERVING: CALORIES 373 PROTEIN (G) 14 CARBS (G) 33 SUGAR (G) 11 FAT (G) 20 SATURATED FAT (G) 10 FIBRE (G) 3.5 SALT (G) 0.9

PASTA & SARDINES

1 tbsp olive oil

1 shallot, finely sliced

2 garlic cloves, finely chopped

1 tbsp tomato purée

zest and juice of 1 lemon

1 tsp red wine vinegar

2 tbsp capers

½ tsp chilli flakes

½ tsp dried oregano

6 cubes of frozen spinach,
    defrosted

400g spaghetti or bucatini

2 x 125g tins of sardines
    (or mackerel), drained

salt and black pepper

To serve

2 tbsp finely chopped parsley

grated Parmesan (optional)

A bowl of pasta always makes us sleepy – whatever the time of day. This makes a good store cupboard dish, as it uses tinned fish and frozen spinach, but you could include fresh spinach instead if you prefer. Just wilt about 100g into the other ingredients before adding the pasta.

Heat the oil in a large sauté pan. Add the shallot and cook gently over a medium heat until softened and starting to brown. Add the garlic and cook for another couple of minutes, then stir in the tomato purée. Stir until the aroma of the tomato purée deepens.

Add the lemon zest and juice, red wine vinegar, capers, chilli flakes and oregano. Stir to combine, then add the spinach. Season with salt and pepper.

Meanwhile, cook the pasta in plenty of boiling, salted water according to the packet instructions. Reserve a ladleful of the cooking water and drain.

Add the pasta to the pan of sauce and toss to coat. Add some of the cooking liquid if the contents of the pan look a bit dry. Break up the fish and carefully toss it through the pasta, then cover the pan with a lid and leave for a minute to warm through.

Serve topped with chopped parsley and grated Parmesan, if using.

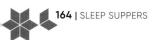

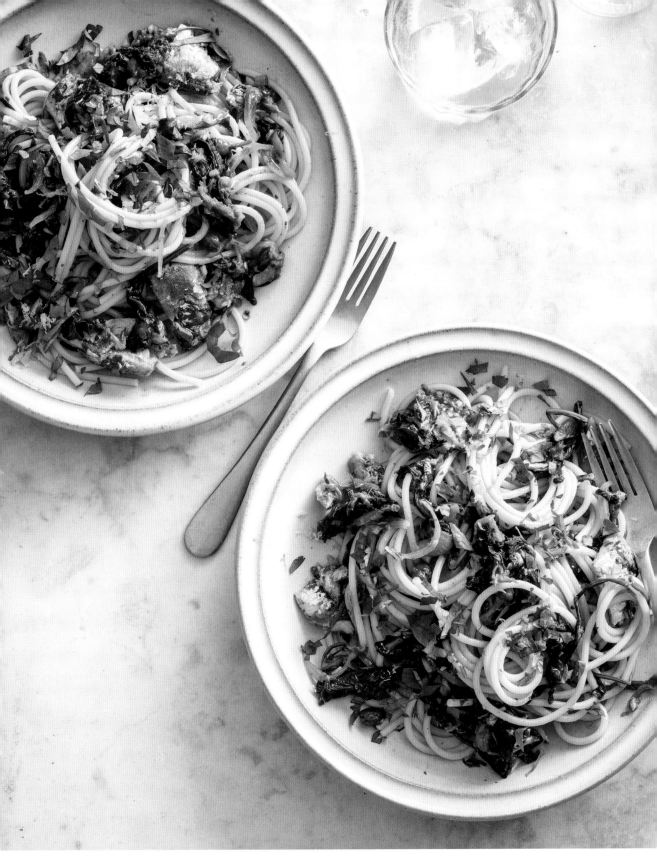

INFO PER SERVING: CALORIES 527 PROTEIN (G) 27 CARBS (G) 73 SUGAR (G) 3 FAT (G) 12.5 SATURATED FAT (G) 2.5 FIBRE (G) 6 SALT (G) 0.7

1 tbsp olive oil

4 little gem lettuces, halved lengthways

15g butter

3 leeks, sliced into rounds

2 garlic cloves, finely chopped

leaves from a small thyme sprig

leaves from a tarragon sprig, finely chopped

100ml white wine

100ml vegetable or chicken stock

300g frozen peas, defrosted

150g ham, diced

50ml crème fraiche

salt and black pepper

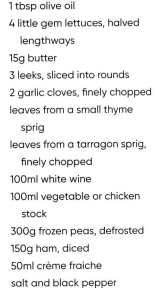

BRAISED LETTUCE WITH LEEKS, PEAS & HAM

Lettuce sent Peter Rabbit off to sleep and we find it works for us too. There's something incredibly soothing about this recipe and it's a great one-pot wonder. The ham adds flavour and it does work well with the pea and leeks, but the dish is still great without if you prefer a vegetarian supper.

Heat the olive oil in a large, lidded sauté pan. Add the little gems, cut-side down, and cook them until well browned. Flip them over and cook for another minute.

Remove the little gems from the pan and set them aside. Melt the butter in the pan and add the leeks. Stir to coat them and cook over a gentle heat for about 5 minutes, then add the garlic, thyme and tarragon.

Put the little gems back in the pan, pour in the wine and bring to the boil. Add the stock, peas and ham, season with salt and pepper, then cover the pan with a lid and simmer for about 15 minutes. Remove the lid and simmer for another 5 minutes until the leeks and little gems are tender.

Add the crème fraiche and swirl it in the pan until it has melted around the vegetables and warmed through. Serve immediately.

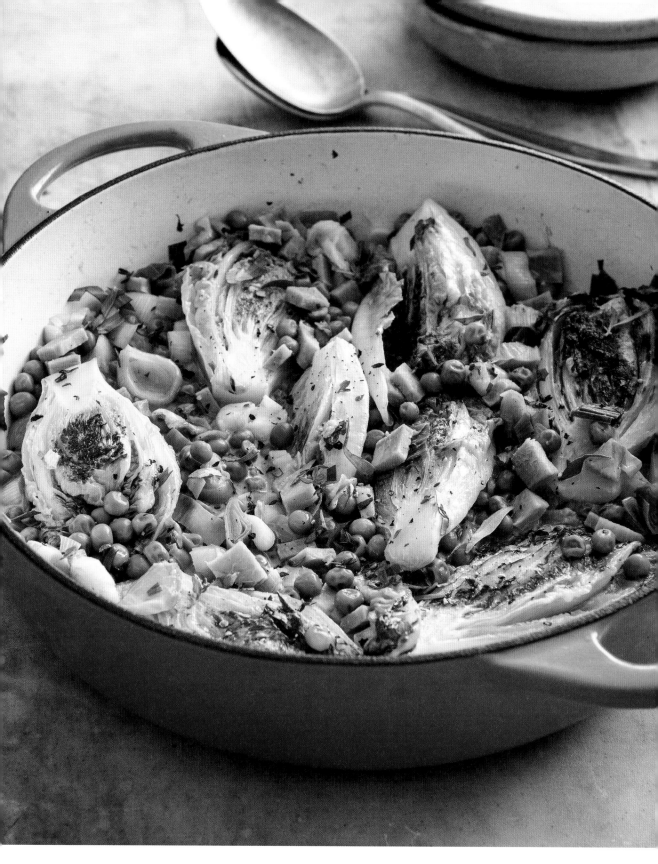

INFO PER SERVING: CALORIES 280   PROTEIN (G) 16   CARBS (G) 13   SUGAR (G) 6   FAT (G) 14   SATURATED FAT (G) 7   FIBRE (G) 9   SALT (G) 0.9

Serves: **4**

 Prep: **15 minutes**

Cooking time: **about 30 minutes**

TURKEY MEATBALLS WITH PASTA

Meatballs

400g turkey or chicken mince

75g fresh breadcrumbs

1 tsp dried oregano

rasp of nutmeg

1 garlic clove, crushed

1 tarragon sprig, leaves
finely chopped

1 egg

salt and black pepper

Pasta and sauce

400g long pasta (tagliatelle,
linguine or spaghetti)

1 tbsp olive oil

1 onion, finely chopped

2 garlic cloves, finely chopped

1 tarragon sprig, leaves
finely chopped

zest of 1 lemon

200ml crème fraiche

To garnish (optional)

freshly grated lemon zest

rasp of nutmeg

a few chilli flakes

freshly grated Parmesan

Turkey is a good source of protein, not too high in fat and said to help sleep by aiding the production of melatonin. Serve these meatballs on a nice bed of pasta and we think you'll agree this is a real keeper. The creamy sauce is delicious and very comforting, but if you're concerned about the fat content, you could use half-fat crème fraiche.

First make the meatballs. Preheat the oven to 200°C/Fan 180°C/Fan 6 and line a baking tray with parchment. Put the mince in a bowl and add all the remaining meatball ingredients, along with plenty of salt and pepper. Mix thoroughly until the mixture becomes less tacky (the easiest thing to do is to knead it with your hands), then form it into 24 small balls. Place these on the baking tray and bake for about 10 minutes until just cooked through.

Cook the pasta in boiling, salted water, according to the packet instructions. Drain, reserving a little of the cooking liquid.

Meanwhile, heat the olive oil in a large sauté pan. Add the onion and cook until soft and translucent, then add the garlic, tarragon and lemon zest. Stir in the crème fraiche and add the meatballs to the sauce. Season with salt and pepper. Loosen the sauce with a ladleful of the cooking liquid and leave to simmer for 5 minutes.

Serve the meatballs and sauce ladled over the pasta with any of the garnishes.

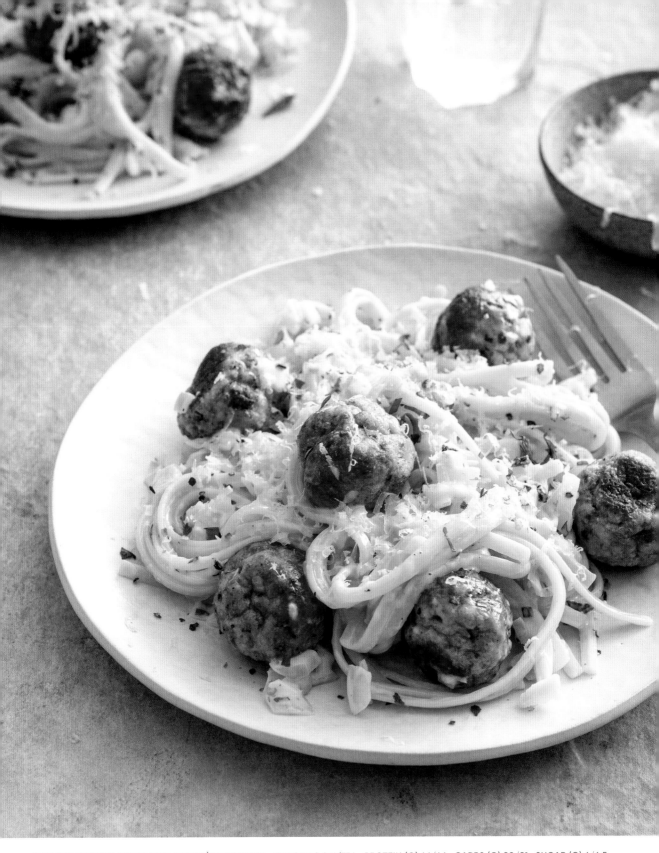

INFO PER SERVING/WITH HALF-FAT CRÈME FRAICHE: CALORIES 861/754   PROTEIN (G) 46/46   CARBS (G) 90/91   SUGAR (G) 6/6.5

FAT (G) 34/21   SATURATED FAT (G) 17/8.5   FIBRE (G) 6/6   SALT (G) 0.5/0.5

BEDTIME SNACKS

GINGERY OAT BISCUITS

Makes: **24**

Prep: **15 minutes**

Cooking time: **15 minutes**

150g wholemeal flour
50g porridge oats
1 tbsp ground ginger
½ tsp bicarbonate of soda
pinch of salt
75g honey
50g butter
75g light brown soft sugar
1 egg yolk

These are a slightly more robust gingernut – made with wholemeal flour and oats to add fibre and with honey instead of the usual golden syrup. Ideal for dunking into your bedtime milky drink.

Preheat the oven to 190°C/Fan 170°C/Gas 5 and line 2 baking trays with baking parchment. Put the flour, oats, ginger and bicarb in a bowl and add a generous pinch of salt. Mix together.

Melt the honey and butter together in a saucepan. Remove from the heat and leave to stand for a couple of minutes, then beat in the sugar and the egg yolk. Fold in the dry ingredients – you will end up with a soft dough that will firm up as it cools and will easily roll into balls.

Divide the mixture into 24 walnut-sized balls, place them on the baking trays and bake them in the oven for 12–15 minutes. The biscuits are ready when they have browned round the edges and puffed up. Remove them from the oven and leave to cool on the baking trays. The biscuits will still be very soft but will subside and set to a crunchy texture. Once they're cool, transfer them to an airtight tin.

SPICED HOT CHOCOLATE

Serves: **2**

Prep: **2 minutes**

Cooking time: **5 minutes**

500ml milk
2 tbsp cocoa powder
pinches of cinnamon, allspice, ginger
pinch of chilli (optional)
pinch of salt
25g dark chocolate, broken up
1–2 tsp honey

A milky drink is always soothing at bedtime and we like to enliven our hot chocolate with a hint of spice and some dark chocolate as well as cocoa powder. If you prefer a milder drink, leave out the dark chocolate.

Put 50ml of the milk in a cup, whisk in the cocoa powder, spices and chilli, if using, and add a pinch of salt. Heat the remaining milk in a saucepan. When the milk is close to boiling point, pour some of it over the contents of your cup. Whisk together and pour everything back into the saucepan.

Add the dark chocolate, if using, and a teaspoon of honey. Stir until the chocolate and honey have dissolved into the milk, then taste and add more honey if you like. Whisk until frothy and piping hot, then divide between 2 mugs.

Serves: **2**

Prep: **1 minute**

Cooking time: **5 minutes**

500ml milk (any sort)

50g malt extract

MALTED MILK

Simply stir some malt extract into hot milk and you have a wonderfully comforting drink that will send you off to bed feeling very happy.

Put the milk and malt extract in a saucepan and heat gently, whisking constantly, until the malt has dissolved into the milk, turning it a rich, biscuity colour. Continue to heat until the milk is just coming up the boil, then divide between 2 mugs.

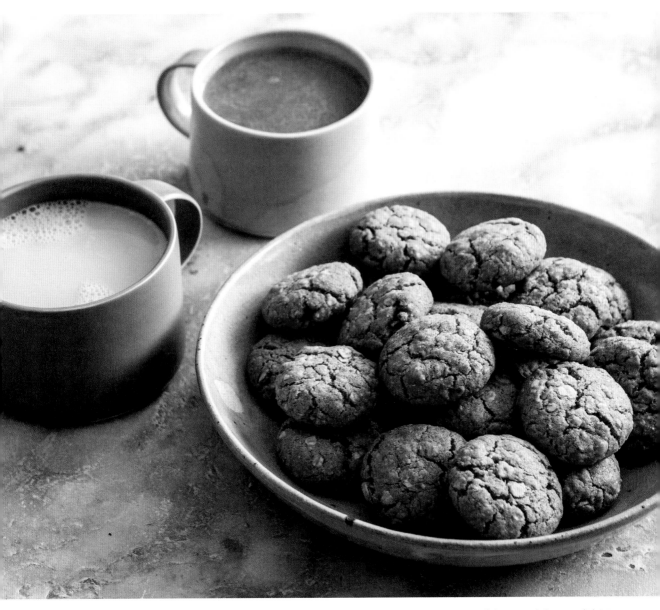

INFO PER BISCUIT: CALORIES 71 PROTEIN (G) 1 CARBS (G) 11 SUGAR (G) 5.5 FAT (G) 2 SATURATED FAT (G) 1 FIBRE (G) 1 SALT (G) 0.1

INFO PER SERVING HOT CHOCOLATE/MALTED MILK: CALORIES 266/192 PROTEIN (G) 12.5/10 CARBS (G) 28/29 SUGAR (G) 26/29

FAT (G) 11/4 SATURATED FAT (G) 7/3 FIBRE (G) 3/0 SALT (G) 0.8/0.2

MILK PUDDINGS

2 egg yolks
2 tbsp cornflour
¼ tsp ground cinnamon
¼ tsp ground allspice
pinch of salt
400ml whole milk
50ml single cream
½ tsp vanilla extract
100ml maple syrup

To serve
pinches of cinnamon
   or cocoa powder

These little bowls of loveliness remind us both of our childhood and are like a comforting hug at end of the end of the day.

Put the egg yolks, cornflour and spices into a bowl with a pinch of salt. Whisk together until well combined.

Put the milk, cream, vanilla extract and maple syrup into a saucepan and heat almost to boiling point. Remove the pan from the heat, then pour the mixture from a height over the egg and cornflour, whisking constantly as you do so.

Pour the mixture back into the saucepan and place over a very low heat. Cook, stirring constantly, until the mixture thickens and starts forming large bubbles.

Pour the mixture through a sieve into a container and cover with lightly oiled plastic wrap. Make sure the plastic wrap is touching the surface of the mixture to prevent a skin from forming. When the pudding has cooled to room temperature, transfer it to the fridge and chill for several hours.

Just before you are ready to serve, whisk the pudding thoroughly, then divide between 4 small bowls or glasses. Sprinkle with a pinch of cinnamon or cocoa powder before serving.

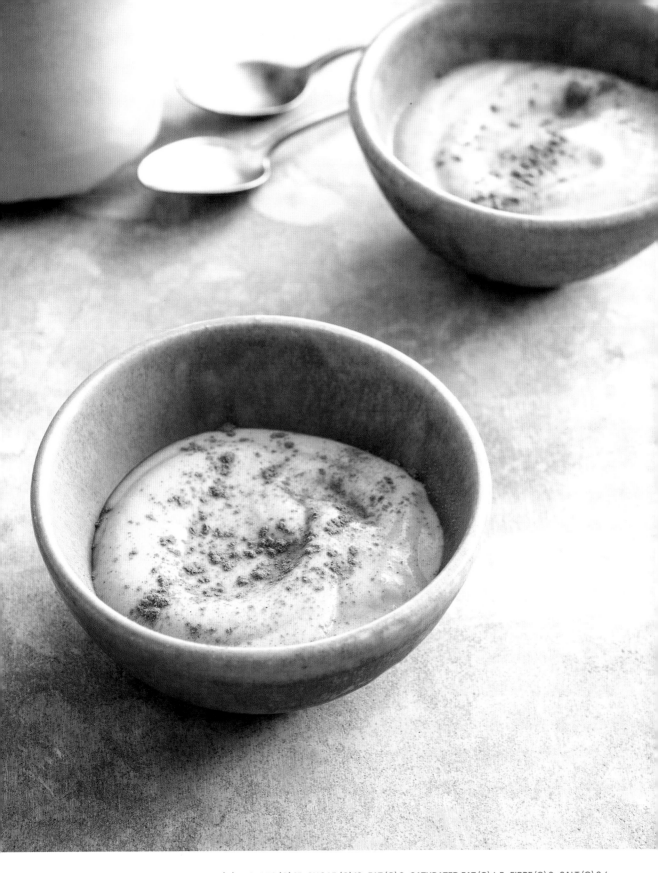

INFO PER SERVING: CALORIES 210   PROTEIN (G) 5   CARBS (G) 27   SUGAR (G) 19   FAT (G) 9   SATURATED FAT (G) 4.5   FIBRE (G) 0   SALT (G) 0.4

125g wholemeal flour
pinch of salt
1 egg
275ml whole milk
vegetable oil

Cherry sauce
400g pitted cherries,
    fresh or frozen
150ml fruit juice
1 tbsp caster sugar
½ tsp ground cinnamon
1 tbsp cornflour
squeeze of lemon

To serve (optional)
crème fraiche or ice cream

PANCAKES WITH CHERRY SAUCE

There are some studies that suggest cherries and cherry juice are good for promoting sleep and we're happy to go along with that and enjoy these fab pancakes. We've kept the sugar and flour to a minimum, so these are reasonably healthy.

First make the pancake batter. Put the flour in a bowl with a pinch of salt and whisk, then make a well in the centre and add the egg. Break up the egg and work it into the flour until you have incorporated most of it into a thick paste. Add some of the milk, gradually to begin with, whisking to keep the mixture lump free. When you have a thick batter, add the rest of the milk. Alternatively, put everything in a blender and pulse – don't overdo it though, as you don't want the mixture to be aerated. Leave the batter to stand for half an hour.

For the cherry sauce, put the cherries in a saucepan with the fruit juice, sugar and cinnamon. Heat gently to dissolve the sugar, briefly bring to the boil, then turn the heat down to a simmer. Mix the cornflour with a little cold water, add about two-thirds of this mixture to the cherries and stir constantly for a few minutes. If the sauce still seems quite runny, add the rest of the cornflour mixture to the pan and stir until the sauce thickens. Add a squeeze of lemon juice.

Lightly oil a crêpe pan or frying pan and place it over a medium-high heat until hot. Pour a ladleful of the batter into the pan, swirling it around so it coats the base completely. When the pancake has completely set on one side, use a palette knife to loosen it, then flip it over and cook it for another minute. Repeat with the remaining batter to make 8 pancakes.

Serve the pancakes warm, filled with spoonfuls of the cherry sauce and with crème fraiche or ice cream on the side, if you like.

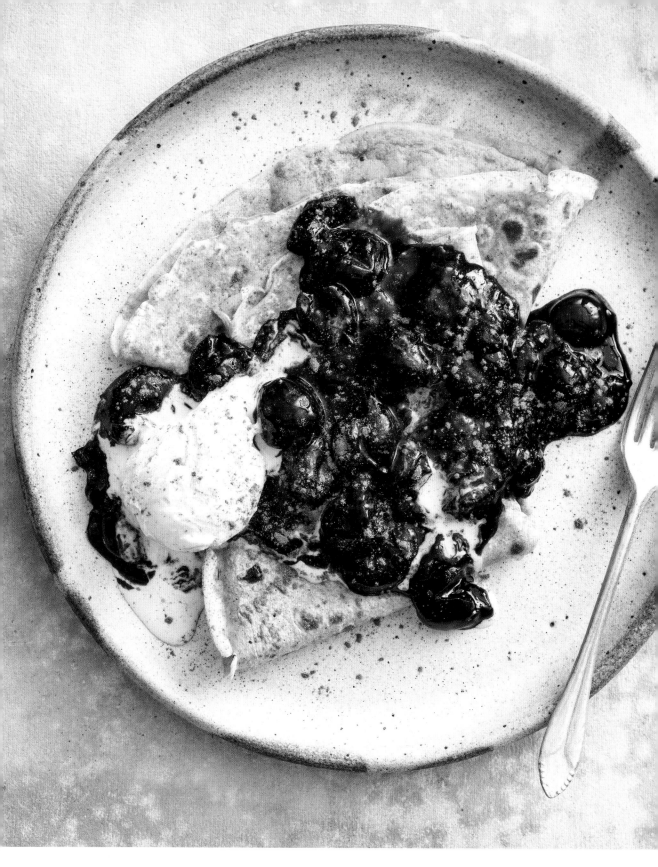

INFO PER SERVING: CALORIES 292   PROTEIN (G) 9   CARBS (G) 45   SUGAR (G) 21   FAT (G) 7   SATURATED FAT (G) 2   FIBRE (G) 4.5   SALT (G) 0.4

Makes: **12 slices**   Prep: **15 minutes**   Cooking time: **35–40 minutes**

oil, for greasing

200g wholemeal flour

2 tsp baking powder

1 tbsp ground ginger, plus extra for sprinkling

½ tsp ground cinnamon

pinch of salt

100g butter, softened

125g caster sugar

3 eggs

100g plain yoghurt

2 pears, cored and each cut into 8 wedges

1 (heaped) tsp honey

PEAR & GINGER UPSIDE-DOWN CAKE

Upside-down cakes are usually caramelised with butter and sugar, but in this recipe we just finish the cake with a light brush of honey. We have to admit that this cake doesn't necessarily contain sleep-friendly ingredients but we do both love a slice of something sweet and tasty in the evening. Sends us off to bed happy!

Preheat the oven to 180°C/Fan 160°C/Gas 4. Lightly oil a deep 20cm cake tin and line it with baking parchment.

Put the flour, baking powder and spices into a bowl with a generous pinch of salt and mix thoroughly.

Beat the butter and sugar together until soft and aerated. Add an egg with a couple of tablespoons of the flour mixture and mix, then repeat with the remaining eggs and further tablespoons of flour. Fold in the rest of the flour followed by the yoghurt. The mixture should have a very reluctant dropping consistency.

Arrange the pears in the base of the tin and spoon the cake batter over them. Bake in the oven for about 35–40 minutes until the cake is well risen and golden and a skewer inserted into the cake comes out clean.

Turn the cake out on to a cooling rack. Melt the honey and brush it over the cake, then sprinkle with a little ground ginger. Leave to cool, then store in an airtight tin.

Tip: You could brush the cake with pear or apricot jam instead of honey, if you like. Or if you happen to have some stem ginger syrup handy that would work a treat.

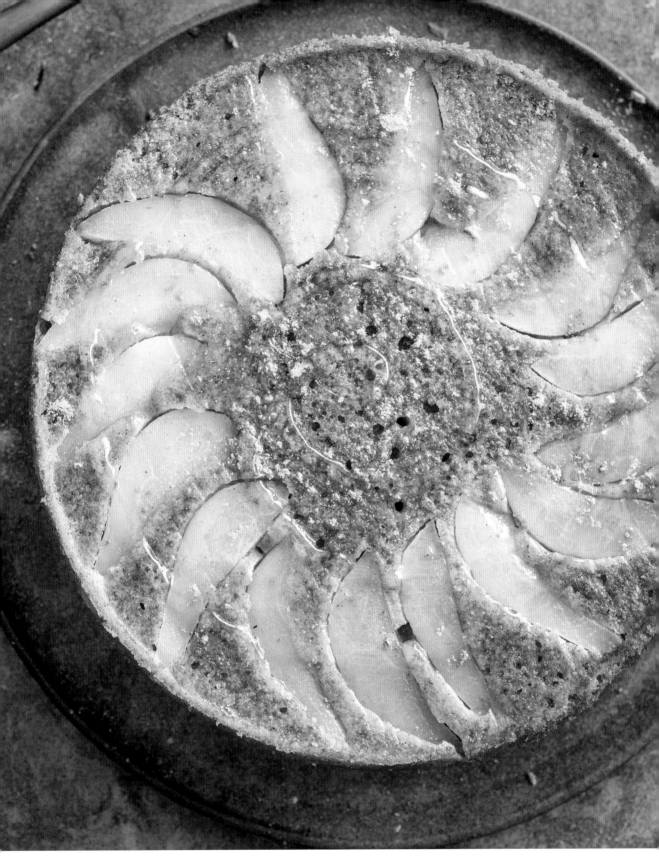

INFO PER SLICE: CALORIES 310   PROTEIN (G) 7   CARBS (G) 38   SUGAR (G) 22   FAT (G) 13   SATURATED FAT (G) 7   FIBRE (G) 3.5   SALT (G) 0.8

4 ripe bananas, cut in half
    lengthways, unpeeled
generous pinch of ground
    cinnamon
generous pinch of ground
    cardamom
zest and juice of 1 lime
25g walnuts, finely chopped
1 tbsp honey
20g dark chocolate

To serve
crème fraiche, Greek yoghurt
    or frozen yoghurt

BAKED BANANAS WITH WALNUTS

Bananas and walnuts are both highly nutritious foods and contain sleep-promoting ingredients, such as tryptophan and magnesium. They make a delicious evening snack, which will help to sustain you through the night. Very simple, very lightly spiced.

Preheat the oven to 200°C/Fan 180°C/Gas 6.

Arrange the bananas in a roasting tin or an ovenproof dish. Sprinkle over the cinnamon, cardamom, lime zest and juice and the nuts. Cover the dish with foil and bake the bananas for about 15 minutes until they are very soft and tender.

Arrange the bananas on 4 plates, skins still on. Drizzle with honey and grate over the chocolate. Serve with dollops of crème fraiche or yoghurt. To eat, scoop the soft flesh out of the banana skins.

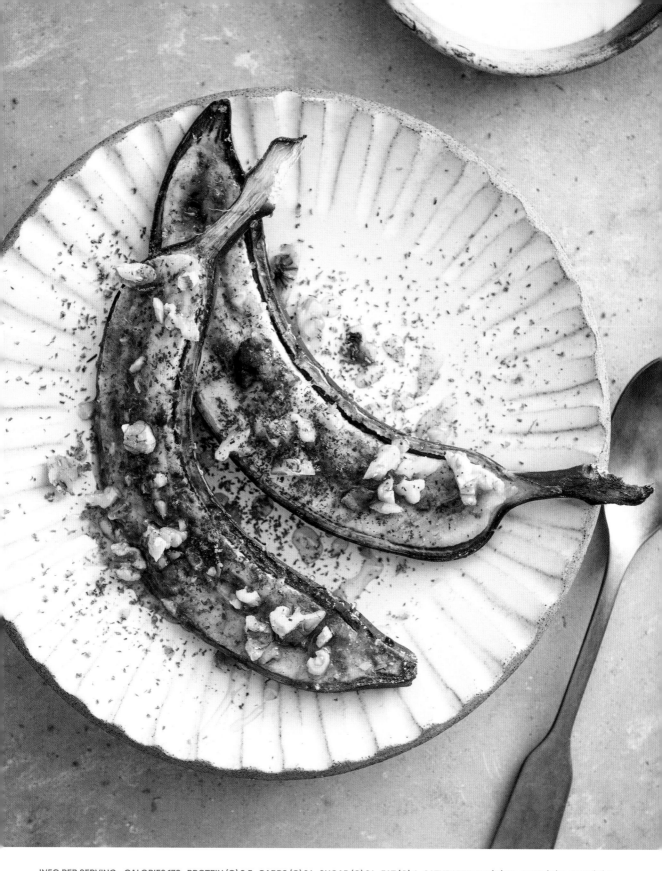

INFO PER SERVING: CALORIES 170 PROTEIN (G) 2.5 CARBS (G) 26 SUGAR (G) 24 FAT (G) 6 SATURATED FAT (G) 1.5 FIBRE (G) 2 SALT (G) 0

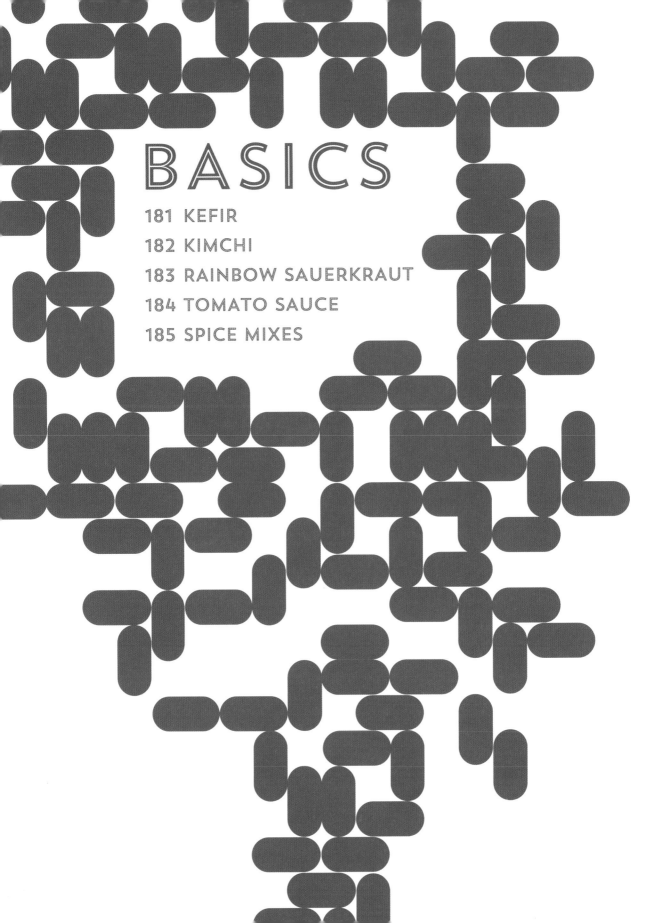

BASICS

KEFIR

10g activated kefir grains
500ml whole milk, preferably
    organic, even better, raw
    organic

We've used kefir in quite a few dishes in this book and although you can buy it, you might like to try making your own – it's easy and cheaper. You have to begin by activating the kefir grains, so follow the instructions provided with them.

Prepare your equipment. You will need a large glass jar – a Kilner one is ideal. You don't need to sterilise it, but do wash it in very hot soapy water and dry it thoroughly.

Put the activated kefir grains in the prepared jar and add the milk. Make sure the jar allows for several centimetres of headroom at the top. If using a Kilner jar of the sort that has a rubber seal, close the lid without the seal. Otherwise, cover the jar with a double layer of muslin or cheesecloth, or a couple of pieces of kitchen paper. Secure this with string or rubber bands.

Leave the jar at room temperature (18°C or above – the warmer it is, the shorter the ferment time) and out of direct sunlight for 18–24 hours. Stir every 6 hours, if you remember. It should thicken in that time, but if it doesn't it will probably be because the temperature has dipped. If it is a hot day, the kefir might ferment in a few hours. When it has thickened, taste and leave it for longer if you want a stronger flavour.

Strain the kefir through a sieve to retrieve the grains. You can start the process again with some or all of the grains (they do grow over time). If you don't want to use them immediately, cover the grains with milk and leave them in the fridge until needed. You can also freeze grains for up to 6 months, then reactivate them.

Store the kefir in the fridge. It will continue to ferment very gently and should be edible for up to a month.

INFO PER 100G: CALORIES 63 PROTEIN (G) 3.4 CARBS (G) 4.5 SUGAR (G) 4.5 FAT (G) 3.5 SATURATED FAT (G) 2.5 FIBRE (G) 0 SALT (G) TRACE

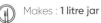
400g kale or 200g kale
  and 200g cabbage

1 large carrot, grated
  or cut into matchsticks

1 large leek, finely sliced
  into rounds

100g radishes, finely sliced

20g sea salt

spring or filtered water

Paste

1–3 tsp chilli powder, to taste

1 tbsp sweet paprika

1 tsp honey

10g root ginger, grated

2 garlic cloves, crushed

1 small piece of fresh turmeric
  root, grated or 1 tsp ground
  turmeric

1 tsp mustard seeds

2 tbsp fish sauce or soy sauce

KIMCHI

Fermented vegetables are reckoned to be really good for your gut and what's good for your gut is good for you. You can buy kimchi in supermarkets, but it's even better if you make it yourself.

First prepare a 1-litre jar. To sterilise it, put it through a hot dishwasher cycle or wash it in hot, soapy water, then rinse it thoroughly and leave to dry in a low oven. Make sure the jar is completely dry before filling.

Shred the kale across the stem or remove the stems and keep the leaves in long strips. If using cabbage as well, shred it finely. Put the kale or kale and cabbage in a bowl with the carrot, leek and radishes. Sprinkle over the salt and rub it into the vegetables until they start to release liquid – it will start with a few droplets of water appearing on the surface. Cover with a plate and weigh the plate down with tins. Leave the vegetables to stand for at least 2 hours, then drain – quite a bit of liquid will have come out of them. Rinse the vegetables with the spring or filtered water, then taste for saltiness. If they're still too salty, rinse again and drain thoroughly.

Mix all the paste ingredients together and pour the paste over the vegetables. Stir to combine, then pack everything into your prepared jar, pushing it all down to make sure there are no air pockets. Seal and leave it somewhere cool and dark for 24 hours.

Remove the lid and press everything down again, then reseal and leave for another 24 hours. You should start to see small bubbles appear on the surface and the kimchi should smell pleasantly sour. At this point, you can put the jar in the fridge or leave it fermenting at room temperature for up to 2 weeks, tasting it daily until it has the flavour you like. Once you put it in the fridge it will keep fermenting and improving in flavour, but the process will slow down considerably.

The kimchi will keep in the fridge indefinitely.

INFO PER 100G: CALORIES 38   PROTEIN (G) 2   CARBS (G) 3.5   SUGAR (G) 3.5   FAT (G) 1   SATURATED FAT (G) 0   FIBRE (G) 3   SALT (G) 2.7

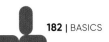

RAINBOW SAUERKRAUT

Like kimchi, this is great for gut health and makes a delicious side dish or snack.

Wash 2 and sterilise 2 large wide-rimmed preserving jars (see opposite) and dry them really thoroughly.

Shred the cabbages and all the other vegetables as finely as you can. The root vegetables can be grated or cut into matchstick strips. Put them all in a large bowl. Add the herbs, but be sparing, as they will carry a lot of flavour. Add the sea salt and rub it into the vegetables until they start to give out liquid – droplets will start to appear on the surface – and you'll feel the texture change. Keep massaging until the cabbage looks wet and is sitting in a pool of water. If it's resistant, you can weigh it down and leave it to stand for an hour.

Stir in the mustard seeds and turmeric, then pack the vegetables into the jars, pressing them down as much as possible to make sure there are no air bubbles. You'll need enough room at the top of each jar to weigh the veg down, so don't fill them more than three-quarters full.

Divide any liquid left in the bowl between the jars. If it doesn't quite cover the vegetables, add a little filtered or spring water. Weigh down the vegetables with special glass weights or use plastic bags filled with water. Or if there's room, you can use a couple of shallow ramekins. Make sure that all the vegetables are sitting below the surface of the liquid, as it's important that they don't come into contact with the air. Seal the jars.

Leave them somewhere cool and dark for several days, checking every day and loosening the lid every day to make sure the build-up of gases within the jars is released. You should start to see small air bubbles appear after 24 hours. Taste the sauerkraut after 4 or 5 days. If you are happy with what should be a pleasantly sour flavour, remove the weights and transfer the jars to the fridge. The sauerkraut will keep fermenting at a much slower rate. Start eating it immediately or leave it for up to several months. Once opened, eat within a few weeks.

½ red cabbage, about 250g

½ white or green pointed cabbage, about 250g

400g mixed vegetables (carrots, red pepper, beetroots, rainbow chard, kale, leek, celeriac, radishes, turnips, garlic)

a few fresh herb sprigs (parsley, mint, coriander, thyme, dill), finely chopped

1 tbsp sea salt

1 tsp mustard seeds

1 tbsp grated fresh turmeric root or 1 tsp ground

spring or filtered water

INFO PER 100G: CALORIES 31   PROTEIN (G) 1   CARBS (G) 4.5   SUGAR (G) 4   FAT (G) 0   SATURATED FAT (G) 0   FIBRE (G) 3   SALT (G) 1.6

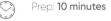
3 tbsp olive oil

1 onion, very finely chopped

4 garlic cloves, very finely
    chopped

2 x 400g cans of tomatoes

1 tsp dried oregano or 1 fresh
    oregano sprig, left whole

basil leaves

sea salt and black pepper

TOMATO SAUCE

This is a good basic tomato sauce to serve with the meatless meatloaf on page 102 or with pasta. Make a double quantity and put some in the freezer for a quick supper when you're busy.

Heat the olive oil in a large saucepan. Add the onion and sprinkle with salt, then cook gently over a low heat until very soft and translucent. Turn up the heat slightly, add the garlic and continue to cook for a couple of minutes. Add the tomatoes and oregano, then season again with salt and pepper.

Bring the sauce to the boil, then turn the heat down to a simmer and cover the pan. Cook for about half an hour, then remove the lid and continue to simmer until the sauce has reduced by just under about a third.

Add a few basil leaves and leave to simmer for another few minutes, just to infuse a little flavour, then remove the basil and the whole oregano sprig, if used. Remove the pan from the heat.

The sauce will keep in the fridge for up to a week and can also be frozen in portions.

INFO PER 100G: CALORIES 190 PROTEIN (G) 1.5 CARBS (G) 7 SUGAR (G) 4.5 FAT (G) 17 SATURATED FAT (G) 2.5 FIBRE (G) 2 SALT (G) TRACE

SPICE MIXES

You can buy spice mixes to use for the recipes in this book, but it's fun to make your own and they'll be even tastier. Give these a try.

For each spice mix, add the spices to a bowl and mix well. Store in an airtight jar.

Tagine spice mix

1 tsp ground cumin

1 tsp ground coriander

1 tsp ground ginger

½ tsp ground cinnamon

½ tsp ground cardamom

½ tsp ground turmeric

½ tsp ground allspice

Cajun spice mix

1 tbsp salt

1 tbsp smoked paprika

1 tbsp garlic powder

1 tbsp onion powder

2 tsp dried oregano

1 tsp dried thyme

1 tsp ground black pepper

1 tsp cayenne

Fajitas spice mix

1 tbsp ground cumin

1 tbsp medium chilli powder

1 tsp ground allspice

1 tsp ground cinnamon

1 tsp sweet smoked paprika

1 tsp dried oregano

1 tsp garlic powder

1 tsp onion powder/granules

INDEX

THANK YOU ALL SO MUCH

This has been a very special book for us and we've made it with the help of some very special people.

First off, mega thanks to our fantastic book team – Catherine Phipps, who has the most incredible food knowledge, Andrew Hayes-Watkins, who has the ability to photograph not only a chicken but us two turkeys as well, Lucie Stericker, who creates our beautiful books, Jinny Johnson, who makes sense of everything, Lola Milne and Hattie Baker, who cook our delicious food and style it so elegantly, and Rachel Vere, who puts the pots and plates together with great style. And to Elise See Tai for proofreading and Vicki Robinson for compiling the index. Also, huge thanks to Fiona Hunter who guided us through the minefields of nutritional knowledge. We've all learned a lot from Fiona and we hope you will too.

As always, thanks to the people at Orion for all their enthusiasm and support – Anna Valentine, Vicky Eribo, Jess Hart, Virgina Woolstencroft, Alainna Hadjigeorgiou, Lynsey Sutherland, Helena Fouracre, Jennifer Wilson and Simon Walsh.

And love and thanks to the wonderful people at ITG, our management – Nicola Ibison, Roland Carreras and Tasha Hall – and to Barrie Simpson, webmaster, and Iza Orzac, social media star.

Last, but never least, thanks to François Gandolfi and all at Southshore, and to Max Gogerty and Catherine Catton
at good old auntie Beeb.

You're all amazing!

Love Si and Dave

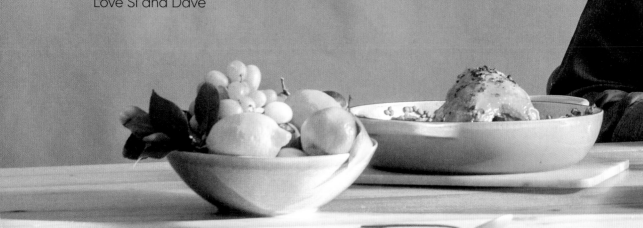

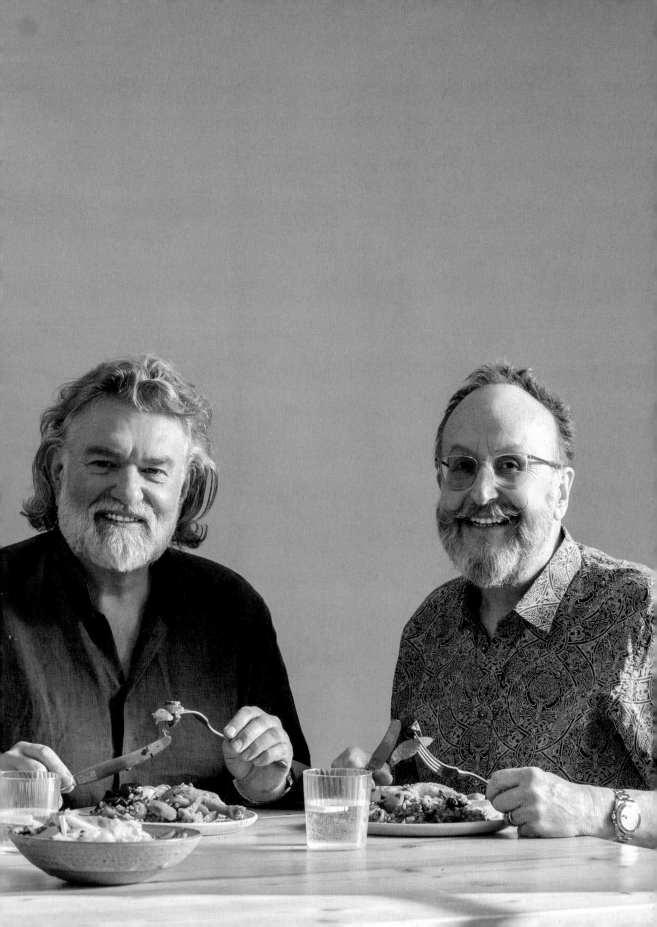

DEDICATION

We'd like to dedicate this book to all our friends, family and colleagues who've given so much amazing support through a difficult time for us both. We hope this book helps you and all our readers stay healthy. In the words of Mr Spock: 'Live long and prosper'.

First published in Great Britain in 2023 by Seven Dials,
an imprint of The Orion Publishing Group Ltd
Carmelite House, 50 Victoria Embankment
London EC4Y 0DZ

An Hachette UK Company

10 9 8 7 6 5 4 3 2 1

ISBN (Hardback) 978 1 3996 0028 6
ISBN (eBook) 978 1 3996 0029 3

Publisher: Vicky Eribo
Recipe consultant: Catherine Phipps
Photography: Andrew Hayes-Watkins
Design and art direction: Lucie Stericker, Studio 7:15
Editor: Jinny Johnson
Food stylist: Lola Milne

Origination by F1 Colour Ltd, London
Printed in Italy by Printer Trento Srl

Food stylist's assistant: Hattie Baker
Prop stylist: Rachel Vere
Proofreader: Elise See Tai
Indexer: Vicki Robinson
Production manager: Simon Walsh
Nutritional consultant: Fiona Hunter, Bsc (Hons) Nutrition, Dip Dietetics

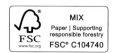

MIX
Paper | Supporting responsible forestry
FSC® C104740
www.fsc.org

www.orionbooks.co.uk